Don't Drink A1 Milk !!

The Type A1/A2 milk issue

and the BCM-7 peptide

…. *the devil in the milk*

Don't Drink A1 Milk !!

The Type A1/A2 milk issue and the BCM-7 peptide
.... *the devil in the milk*

Brent Bateman

Bsc, Msc Human Nutrition

Another book in the series
The Nutrition Factor: A Bold New Perspective

ISBN 978-0-9796987-3-6

DEDICATION

This expose' is dedicated to the ongoing struggle to improve our human health.

True progress in human health can sometimes be thwarted by the self-interest of big business or by government agencies being subservient to those interests, or by corrupt and mischievous politics, or stagnation due to unjustified complacency.

The result is that the final responsibility often falls on the shoulders of you and I ... the general public ... the consumers. And it is us who must ultimately protest and demand transparency, integrity, and courage from those who control our health and welfare.

More specifically, this treatise is dedicated to promoting awareness and knowledge of the health hazards of consuming Type A1 cow's milk; and prompting the dairy industry, the various governments, and the scientific community to confront this health risk and to take remedial action.

FOREWORD

The issue ... the evidence ... the implications ... and a call for accountability and action !!

This expose' is written as a follow-up to the author's recently published *MILK ... to drink, or not to drink ??* Whereas *MILK* presented an objective overview of the full spectrum of the pros and cons of consuming cow's milk as a food choice for humans, this treatise is directed specifically at the Type A1 and Type A2 milk issue and the casomorphin peptide, BCM-7 ... *the devil in the milk.*

We now know that the beta-casein protein in Type A1 milk can generate the BCM-7 peptide, which is highly bioactive and is hypothesized to be a causative factor in the onset of a number of disease conditions. It can theoretically attach itself to the insulin-producing beta cells in the pancreas, prompting an autoimmune response that can destroy the beta cells, thereby leading to diabetes. The BCM-7 molecule is a strong oxidant, and can oxidize LDL cholesterol, contributing to the build-up of plague in the arteries, or atherosclerosis. It is also a powerful morphine-like opiate that can pass through the *blood-brain barrier* and create havoc with normal brain function, promoting neurological disorders such as schizophrenia and autism.

The author explores the evidence in Chapter Two, demonstrating that the research findings, although *not yet* conclusive in a strict scientific sense, are both credible and compelling, and cannot be ignored.

The 'problem' addressed in Chapter Three is separated into two parts: (a) the potential health hazard of drinking Type A1 milk, based on our new knowledge, and (b) the attempt by the dairy industry *and* various government regulatory and food safety agencies to discredit the scientific evidence and to suppress awareness of the potential health risk. The author suggests that *if* there is truly a potential health risk associated with consuming Type A1 cow's milk, and the government and dairy industry are aware of this potential, then we, the consumers, have been deceived, and *are* being deceived even now, as you read this book.

The most critical part of the message of the expose', then, is an alert, and a call for accountability and action. The author suggests that what is at stake is much more than a simple challenge to the dairy industry ... what is more importantly at stake is our basic health, and that of our children, and of generations to come ... and the increasing millions who are suffering and *will* suffer from diabetes, heart disease, and neurological disorders. He suggests that it may not be so much a matter of what science finally concludes ... although this is extremely important ... it may be more a matter of consumer's being told the truth, being protected, and having a choice. Chapter Four therefore draws attention to the need for additional research, for accountability, and for action.

The author also suggests that there is a genuinely positive side to this issue ... with our new knowledge of the BCM-7 peptide, we may have at our finger tips a key to removing a significant cause of chronic disease and uplifting our human health to an even higher level.

The author has decided to continue the approach initiated in *MILK ... to drink, or* not *to drink ??* by listing the references at the end of each chapter, with comments. The goal is to make it easier for the reader to follow and understand the references and to be able to draw their own conclusions.

This treatise and *MILK* are part of the author's series entitled *The Nutrition Factor: A Bold New Perspective*, in which the author proposes that our 'conventional wisdom' paradigm in nutrition and health care are leading us in the wrong direction ... that a 'paradigm shift' is long over-due, and a 'bold new perspective' is needed. The Appendix outlines this in greater detail.

The appendix also includes a brief overview of the 'scientific method' and a review of the various research-study designs, statistics, and common terms ... presented to assist the reader in understanding the scientific research and conclusions presented in the text.

TABLE OF CONTENTS

Chapter One

INTRODUCTION

The Type A1/A2 Milk Issue and the BCM-7 Peptide ... *the devil in the milk*

We now know that the genetic base of all cow's milk is *not* the same. One critical difference is in the structure and amino acid composition of the beta-casein portion of the milk protein. There are at least fifteen different variants, each determined by the genetic code on the dairy cow's sixth chromosome. Ten of the most common variants are A1, A2, A3, B, C, D, E, F, G, and H, which are usually grouped as either Type A1 or Type A2, based on which amino acid occupies position 67 in the 209 amino acid chain of all beta-casein protein. A *histidine* amino acid at position 67 was the first discovered, and this type was therefore named 'A', and then later 'A1'. It was found that types B, C, F, G, and H also characterized a histidine at position 67. Because most milk production is Type A1, however, all of these variants are commonly grouped as A1. Further investigation showed that the other genetic variants had a *proline* amino acid at position 67, and it was also determined that this was the original, and *normal*, genetic form. Thus, A2, A3, D, and E genetic variations have a proline at position 67. Similar to the case with Type A1, most milk production with the variant characterizing a proline at position 67 is Type A2, and thus the four variants in this group are commonly grouped together as A2.

With a *histidine* at position 67, Type A1 beta-casein digests differently ... the 209 amino acid chain folds at this point, and a seven-amino-acid fragment containing positions 60 through 66 frequently breaks off. Named BCM-7, this peptide has become known as the *devil in the milk*, in reference to the book by this title, written by Dr. Keith Woodford, a New Zealand farm management specialist. This fragment, or peptide, is highly bioactive and can work in various ways to promote disease conditions within humans. It can attach itself to the insulin-producing beta cells in the pancreas, prompting an autoimmune response which can result in the destruction of the beta cells, leading to diabetes. The BCM-7 molecule is a strong oxidant, and can oxidize LDL cholesterol, contributing to the build-up of plague in the arteries, or atherosclerosis, and thus ischemic heart disease. It is also a powerful morphine-like opiate and can pass through the *blood-brain barrier* to interfere with normal brain function and promote neurological disorders such as schizophrenia and autism.

The replacement of a histidine amino acid instead of a proline is thought to be the result of a mutation occurring in the ancestors of the Holstein-Friesian breed of cattle in Europe several thousand years ago. The Holstein-Friesian is the main milk-producing breed in most Western countries. Almost *all* of the milk sold in the United States contains Type A1. Country exceptions include France, Iceland and India, whose native dairy breeds are nearly pure A2 producers.

The world is indebted to Dr. Keith Woodford, who brought together all the research studies and the actions and manipulations of the various players in the unfolding of the fascinating A1/A2 milk and BCM-7 saga … presented in his book *Devil In The Milk*, first published in New Zealand in 2007, followed by a North American edition in 2009. When his book first went on sale in New Zealand and Australia it attracted a great deal of media attention in those two countries, and the New Zealand Food Safety Authority (NZFSA) immediately attempted to discredit the scientific evidence and downplay the significance of the issue. The European Food Safety Authority (EFSA) was asked by the NZFSA to also review the evidence and to determine if a risk assessment and preventive action was warranted. The EFSA report, issued on January 29th, 2009, concluded the following:

"Based on the present review of available scientific literature, a cause-effect relationship between the oral intake of BCM-7 or related peptides and aetiology or course of any suggested non-communicable diseases cannot be established. Consequently, a formal EFSA risk assessment of food-derived peptides is not recommended." (EFSA, 2009)

The report not only concluded that a risk assessment was not warranted, but it curiously failed to recommend further studies or research and at one point even suggested that using public funds for additional study was also not warranted.

The stance taken by the NZFSA and the EFSA is startling, considering the dearth of evidence and the strength of its credibility.

The EFSA review was used by the New Zealand and Australian governments, and various other governments, to discredit and diffuse the issue, presenting an obvious 'heads in the sand' approach. Curiously, the U.S. Food and Drug Administration has not made any comment on the issue … a search of their website turns up zilch.

Dairy farmers in the U.S., Canada, and Europe know little, if anything, about the Type A1/ Type A2 controversy. Ironically, however, Type A2 milk is available on grocery shelves in New Zealand and Australia, thanks to the efforts of A2 Corporation, and New Zealand dairy farmers are quietly converting their herds to A2-only producers.

An Introduction To Cow's Milk

How we came to be the only animal that drinks the milk of other animals

All domestic cattle, and the *cow*, are descended from the ancient primordial ox, or the *auroch*, with the scientific name *Bos primigenius* (first cow). The now-extinct auroch was a truly massive beast, nearly twice the size of the largest modern cow, and with a fierceness equal to that of the lion or bear. Julius Caesar, speaking of rare encounters with the few aurochs remaining in the wild during his era, judged that they were about the size of small elephants, and to be able to kill one immortalized a hunter. (Montgomery, 2004)

So domestication must surely have been a long and challenging process, with the auroch first being hunted in their natural habitat for their meat, hides, and bones, and then later held in captivity and slowly bred over many generations for softer temperaments and smaller size. Domestication to the degree to allow humans to remove milk from their udders did not occur until about 7,000 years ago, and the first cows produced less than one quart of milk per day. Extensive selective breeding, cross-breeding, and the occurrence of mutations over the millennia have greatly modified and expanded that single *Bos primigenius* beginning. There are now about 920 dairy cattle breeds worldwide, which include many indigenous breeds surviving in specific areas. These include several Asian breeds, the *Norske* dairy cow of Iceland, and the *Normande* French cow, all of which are almost pure A2 producers (this observation becomes important in the discussion in the following chapters).

However, most modern-day dairy cattle belong to the humpless sub-species *Bos taurus,* which is further divided into *Bos taurus indicus*, adapted to hot climates, and *Bos taurus taurus*, adapted to cooler climates. Six breeds predominate in the United States and most of the Western countries, which are

4

the Ayrshire, the Brown Swiss, the Guernsey, Jersey, Milking Shorthorn, and the Holstein-Friesian. The Aryshire, originally from Scotland, is known for their hardiness; the small Jersey and Guernsey for the high cream *and* high protein content of their milk; and the familiar black and white Holstein-Friesian is esteemed for its un-matched rate of production. The Holstein-Friesian, originally from Germany, is the predominant breed in the U.S., Europe, and other Western Countries such as New Zealand and Australia. The milk produced by each of the many different breeds varies considerably in content, and the content can also be influenced by feed and local environmental factors.

Milk Production and Consumption

Milk is the opaque white liquid produced by the mammary glands of mammals, and universally provides the primary nutrient source for young mammals before they are able to digest other types of food. The milk of each species is therefore specific for that species. In other words, the make-up of the milk of each animal is different, and reflects the special needs of that species. Humans are the only animal species that consumes the milk of other animals, *and* continues to do so past the infant weaning stage into childhood and adulthood. As an example, calves … the infant young of the cow … suckle their mother's mammary gland only to the age of approximately 3 months, when their weaning period ends. Young calves, once having reached the end of their weaning period, typically refuse the milk of their mothers and seek other foods. It is also noteworthy that the first milk for the newborn calf, 'colostrum', is very different from the milk produced later … it is heavy with extra nutrients and hormones designed to give the newborn calf its needed boost.

Drinking fluid milk in significant quantities did not become common until very recently, relatively speaking. Melanie DuPuis, in her delightful book, *Nature's Perfect Food,* reminds us that drinking fluid cow's milk did not really become popular

5

in America or Europe until the mid-eighteen hundreds, and even then there were several decades of bitter debate over whether or not it was advisable to consume it at all in that form (more about this below).

During our recent history, we humans have consumed the milk of many different animals, depending largely on which animals were available in each geographic area. These include the water buffalo, camel, horse, reindeer, donkey, and yak, plus the goat, sheep, and even the moose. In Russia and Sweden small moose dairies still exist. More recently, we have found that the cross-breed of the cow and the bison also produces large quantities of milk.

And yes, we *do* consume a lot of milk and related dairy products. Northern Europeans consume the highest per capita amounts, with Finland topping the list at 183.9 liters of liquid milk per person per annum, 19.1 kilograms of cheese, and 5.3 kilograms of butter.

It is noteworthy for later discussion that Finland has the highest per capita intake of cow's milk, almost all of its milk is Type A1 or contains Type A1.

Due to population size, however, the U.S. produces the largest amount of cow's milk, with total tonnage reaching 82.5 million tons in 2006 (University of Guelph, 2010).

The average daily production for all conventional dairy cows in the U.S. in 2005 was 26.8 quarts (24.1 liters). The art of milking cows has come a long way.

The Composition of Milk

The following table lists the main constituents of cow's milk, with the range and average (mean) percent content by weight.

Constituent	Range (%)	Mean (%)
Water	85.5 – 89.5	87.0
Total solids	10.5 – 14.5	13.0
Fat	2.5 – 6.0	4.0
Proteins	2.9 – 5.0	3.4
Lactose	3.6 – 5.5	4.8
Minerals	0.6 – 0.9	0.8

Milk is basically a water-based fluid with 'globules' of butterfat, and 'micelles' (small groups of molecules) of protein … both of which combine to form an 'emulsion', or 'colloid'. The complex sugar, lactose, is soluble with the water portion, forming a molecular solution.

Milk fats

Whole milk contains four types of fats: saturated fat (approximately 65% of the total fat), monounsaturated (about 29%), polyunsaturated (3.6%), and cholesterol (0.5%).

Milk carbohydrates (sugars), lactose

Lactose is a disaccharide sugar, made up of equal portions of the simple sugars glucose and galactose. In order for lactose to pass through the small intestine wall membranes it must first be cleaved into glucose and galactose, requiring the enzyme *lactase*. Lactose is the major carbohydrate in almost all animal milks, and most animal infants produce the enzyme lactase during their weaning period, enabling them to digest the milk lactose. However, the production of this enzyme normally declines sharply after the weaning period … for all animals, including humans. Some human populations, or individuals, have adapted or have benefited from a genetic alteration, which enables them to produce lactase after their infant weaning period, even into adulthood. *Not* producing the enzyme lactase after infancy is the *norm*. Most Asian, African, and Native American populations (including central and South America) are lactase deficient after infancy.

7

Nature's Most Perfect Food

Yes ... we have all been indoctrinated since toddler's age of the proverbial goodness of *milk* ... as dear to us as mom and apple pie. We have all chuckled at the milk mustaches sported by celebrities, and have been convinced that we must drink several tall glasses of milk each day if we are to have healthy bones and enough essential protein. After all, as we have all been told countless times, milk is 'nature's most perfect food' !!

The ability to extract and consume the milk from the udders of domesticated animals is suggested to be a positive factor in the evolution of human populations and cultures. Recent studies in anthropology and genetics have shown that the ability to successfully consume the milk of other animals enabled human populations to survive and multiply much more effectively. For example, Dr. Sarah Tishkoff and her team from the University of Maryland have calculated that the ability to use milk as a source of food nutrition may have contributed to population growth as much as ten times, compared with populations which did not consume animal milk. (Wade, 2006)

A Rich Source of Many Nutrients

Cow's milk is a particularly rich source of protein and several vitamins and minerals, most notably calcium and phosphorus. For each of these nutrients a daily intake equivalent to 4 servings would provide between 25 and 100% of the RDA guideline amounts. For example, a single eight-ounce glass of whole milk provides an American adult 14% of their recommended protein intake with 139 kcalories of energy, 25.6% of their daily need for calcium, 27.2 % of their required phosphorous, 31.9% of the B-vitamin, riboflavin, 13.1% of vitamin A, 42.6 % of B-12, 16.9% B-6, and 12.6 % of their omega-3 requirement. (USDA, IOM). It also contains lesser amounts of iron, magnesium, zinc, potassium, sodium, copper, selenium, and manganese, in amounts ranging from 6 to 18% of the RDA with 4 servings.

The efficiency of absorption or the *bioavailability* of the nutrients in milk is thought to be particularly high compared with other food sources. This is especially true for the proteins in milk and the minerals, most noticeably calcium. The reasons are not fully understood, but the presence of lactose and phosphorous is thought to be a contributing reason, plus the observance that milk remains in the stomach and small intestines for a longer time than do most other food substances, thereby allowing absorption to take place more completely.

This extended time factor during digestion is important to keep in mind when considering the absorption of the BCM-7 peptide, which will be discussed in the next chapter.

Protein

The importance of protein in nutrition cannot be understated. In fact, the word 'protein' is derived from the Greek, *proteos,* meaning 'primary', or 'taking place first'.

Proteins in foods become available for use by our human physiologies after they have been broken down into the component amino acids, of which nine are *essential*, or *indispensible* (the ninth, histidine, is essential only for infants). By essential, we mean that if we have zero intake, death will be the eventual outcome. In recent years, however, this definition has been softened to include 'conditionally essential' and 'acquired indispensability'. If a given protein contains all of the nine essential amino acids, it is then considered to be *complete*, although one or more of the amino acids may be in relatively short supply, and therefore can influence the ability of the total to be utilized … these are dubbed *limiting* amino acids.

Protein is utilized in a number of critical roles. These roles include: (a) forming contractile proteins in muscle, including 'actin' and 'myosin'; (b) constructing fibrous proteins such as

9

collagen, elastin, and keratin; (c) creating molecules that act as *enzymes* ... which act as catalysts to change the rate of biochemical reactions; (d) as derivatives to form hormones; (e) forming immunoproteins to assist in the immune system; (f) assisting in the transport of other proteins; (g) to act as a 'buffer' to ameliorate changes in pH (acidity or alkalinity) of the blood and other body tissues; and (h) to conjugate with other nonprotein compounds to form such entities as 'glycoproteins' and 'lipoproteins'.

The major protein in milk is *casein*, which comprises 76 to 86% of the milk protein, and is divided into alpha-casein, beta casein, and gamma casein, with alpha casein being the major portion (60% of the total casein). Alpha casein is further separated into 'alpha-s-casein' and 'k-casein'. Beta-casein comprises approximately 27% of the total casein ... and is comprised of a continuous chain of 209 amino acids. The amino acid sequence varies, however, with at least fifteen known variations in the sequence.

The remaining 14 to 24% of the protein portion in milk is a variety of proteins collectively called 'whey proteins', of which *lactoglobulin* is the most common (7-12% of the total whey proteins). 'Whey' is also the technical term used to describe the conglomerate typically left behind when the caseins coagulate into 'curds'. The whey proteins are typically more water-soluble than the casein proteins, and do not form large structures. They are therefore more easily absorbed, and are considered an exceptionally rich source of amino acids, some of which are less available from other sources.

Reviewing this past section, therefore, it would seem that milk is indeed a food choice rich in nutrients and one could conclude that it is an almost perfect natural food. However ....

Some Arguments Against Milk As A Food For Humans

The Milk Protein Controversy (Prior to the Type A1/A2, BCM-7 Issue)

Interest in the bioactivity of cow's milk protein has prompted scientific research and studies dating back to the 1950s and even before. On the negative side, concern for allergic reactions in infants was a primary issue, and a great deal of research has historically been directed to this problem. It was recognized early on that various amino-acid segments, or peptides, could remain intact even through digestion and that these peptides could be highly bioactive and were sometimes associated with ill-health symptoms in humans, especially infants. Now termed 'Cow's Milk Allergy', or CMA, it is recognized that a number of different peptides could be the source of the problem. According to one well known research group, Crittenden et al (2005), more than 30 individual peptides have been implicated. It is recognized that CMA is separate from reactions caused by lactose intolerance (or lactase insufficiency) and is commonly divided into (a) immunoglobulin E (IgE)-mediated allergy and non-IgE mediated allergy. Estimates of the percent of infants in the U.S. affected by CMA range from a conservative 2% to as high as 6%, and the immunopathological mechanisms remain poorly understood. (Critenden et al, 2005)

On the positive side there has been a surge of scientific inquiry during the past decade, largely sponsored by the dairy industry and commercial infant formula manufacturers, directed at identifying and generating milk derived peptides that exhibit *beneficial* health effects. An excellent review study by Korhonen et al (2006) reveals that a large number of peptides have been identified and studied, and discusses their occurrence in dairy products, their natural and commercial production, and their beneficial metabolic functions. Production can be via three

11

main methodologies: enzymatic hydrolysis, microbial fermentation, and fractionation and enrichment. Beneficial functions include (a) lowering blood pressure, (b) protection against harmful viruses and bacteria, (c) assisting blood clotting, (d) increasing energy and athletic performance, (e) acting as a relaxant and sleep aid, (f) assisting mineral absorption, and (g) preventing dental caries. (Korhonen and Pihlanto, 2006)

However, none of these studies on either the positive or negative nature of milk protein peptides specifically identified or investigated the β-casein seven amino acid sequence 60-66 ... the BCM-7 peptide .... the *devil in the milk*.

It is important to note that the peptides previously identified as having either negative or positive properties contain up to 20 amino acids in their fragment sequence. Despite such a large number of AAs, they have been shown to successfully transport across the intestinal membranes into the blood stream ... although the conditions necessary to do so are not clear. This is important when considering the seven amino acid sequence of the BCM-7 fragment, because it has been argued that this peptide cannot enter the blood stream of normal human adults due to its large size, and therefore cannot play a disruptive role in the onset of diabetes, heart disease, and neurological disorders. This is then a related controversy.

Twelve other arguments against consuming cow's milk

1. Milk was not a food choice for our pre-agriculture ancestors, and it is questionable whether our physiologies are suitably adapted for its consumption.

Milk was not a food choice for ancestral humans ... domestication of the cow sufficient to extract milk from its udder did not take place until about 7,000 years ago, and drinking large quantities of liquid milk did not become popular until much

12

later.   Melanie DuPuis, in her delightful book, *Nature's Perfect Food* (2002), reminds us that drinking fluid cow's milk did not really become popular in America until the mid-eighteen hundreds, and that there were several decades of bitter debate over whether or not it was advisable to drink it at all, even then. Prior to that time most cow's milk was consumed in fermented forms, or as cheese and other products.   Drinking fluid milk 'straight from the cow' became popular primarily as a breast-milk substitute for infants and a beverage for weaned children. Dupuis explains that the historically unprecedented transition from breastfeeding to using cow's milk as a substitute was the result of a major shift during that era in women's perception of themselves and their bodies, plus the effects of urbanization and heightened socio-economic status.   In addition, the availability, convenience, and low cost of milk made it an attractive food option for the rapidly expanding urban populations.   But in those early years fluid milk, especially as it was aggressively produced for the burgeoning urban masses, such as in New York City, was unclean and the source of much ill health.   The medical historian, P.J. Atkins, dubbed cow's milk as it was produced in the mid-eighteen-hundreds as "white poison".   He provides historical evidence that the milk of the time "was heavily contaminated with bacteria and was responsible for spreading a variety of diseases such as scarlet fever and tuberculosis. Infants not wholly breastfed were particularly vulnerable to diarrheal infections as well.   Improvements such as pasteurization and bottling were slow to spread and had little beneficial impact before the 1920s." (Atkins, 1992)

S. Boyd Eaton and Melvin Konner introduced nutritional science to the concept that our physiologies are designed for a lifestyle and food supply that existed prior to the age of agriculture, which began approximately 10,000 years ago. They first published the results of their arduous and meticulous studies in the prestigious *New England Journal of Medicine* in 1985, followed with a book entitled *The Paleolithic Prescription* three

13

years later. Some of their observations and conclusions were truly startling. For example, they noted that with the advent of agriculture humankind's average height dropped six inches, and that the domestication of animals and food plants radically changed the nutrient quality of both food sources. Applied to the case of cow's milk, the question arises as to whether or not our modern-day physiologies are suited to the consumption of this relatively new food. Eaton and Konner suggest that the answer is 'no' … that the consumption of cow's milk is too recent an event for our physiologies to have genetically modified or adapted to accommodate this food, particularly as adults. The prevalence of lactose intolerance among most non-Northern European ethnic groups worldwide would be a supportive case in point for this conclusion. On the other hand, the apparent mutations that occurred among early ancestors of some Northern European populations and at least two early African groups suggest otherwise. What remains clear is that *most* of the world's population remains lactose intolerant as adults.

2. With increased knowledge about our human nutrient needs and improved food composition data, the finding that cow's milk is lacking in many essential nutrients.

Is it possible that 'nature's most perfect food' could be seriously lacking in some essential nutrients? Well, it is not only possible, but it is fact!

Vitamin C

Cow's milk has no vitamin C. The USDA Food Composition Data Base reports that 100 grams of whole cow's milk contains 0.0 milligrams of vitamin C. Is this surprising? What about the vitamin C in cow's food? There is no data for the vitamin C content of field grasses, but the content in lemon grass is 2.6 mg per 100 grams. The two most-used grain feeds are soybean and corn … one hundred grams of raw soybeans contains only 6 mg of vitamin C, and 100 grams of raw sweet corn 6.8 mg. But even the little that is contained in the normal cow's food is apparently not transferred to its milk. This makes sense, however, when it is realized that the cow ... *and* its calf ... produces its own vitamin C. This is one of the curiosities of our human metabolism and a quirk of mother nature. All of the animals in the animal kingdom produce their own vitamin C, except, that is, for a tiny group which include humans, the gorilla and chimpanzee, the guinea pig, fruit bat, and one species of birds. We lack the last enzyme in the vitamin C synthesis pathway, *gulonolactone oxidase* . Yes, we are *that* close to completing the synthesis pathway. (*Advanced Nutrition And Human Metabolism, 2005*) This fact suggests that at one time, earlier in our evolution, our ancestors *did* produce vitamin C, but that a negative mutation prevented the final step. It also suggests that the mutation took hold because our ancestors at that time lived in an environment so abundant in vitamin C that there was no need for us to make our own. Humans, therefore, must obtain this important essential nutrient in our food supply, but not the cow and almost all other animals. And therefore drinking milk cannot help us get any of this essential vitamin.

Vitamin A and D

Milk is touted for its ability to give us the fat soluble vitamins A, especially vitamin D, and also vitamins E and K ... which are contained in the fat part of milk. Vitamin D is normally required for our bodies to absorb and utilize calcium, so it could be considered a critically essential component of milk, or essentially included in the diet, needed to utilize the calcium in milk. However, if the fat in milk is taken out, as with lowfat or skim milk, then these vitamins are taken out as well. An eight-ounce serving of whole milk contains 104 mg of vitamin A, 0.23 mg of vitamin D, 160 mg of vitamin E, and 0.7 mg of vitamin K, but the same serving of lowfat milk (1% fat) provides only 32 mg of vitamin A, 0 mg of vitamin D, 0.02 mg of vitamin E, and 0.23 mg of vitamin K. Even with the case of whole milk, however, these vitamins are not well supplied: one 8-ounce glass of whole milk provides only 13% of your recommended vitamin A intake, 4.5 % vitamin D, 1.1% vitamin E, and 1.7% vitamin K. For lowfat milk these percentages drop to 4.0%, 0.0001%, 0.00001%, and 0.6%, repectively.

Iodine

The amount of iodine in cow's milk, taken from samples worldwide, cannot be detected by normal laboratory methods (Kikuchi, 2008). Most of the modern world's population obtains iodine from iodized salt ... salt that has been treated with iodine. It is therefore added to our customary diets as a fortification, a form of supplementation. The availability of iodine in our environment has been steadily declining. Normally available in the soil, it has been steadily depleted in most areas of the world, especially in high altitude areas, having been evaporated into the air because of its high volatility, or washed to the sea. Plants that grow in the ocean, such as seaweed and kelp, have therefore been good sources of iodine ... but recent reports and measurements indicate that even the availability of iodine in the coastal seas has been declining. In addition, many cultures in the world do not use iodized salt, and therefore are at risk of iodine deficiency. It is considered one of the four major nutrient deficiencies in the developing world, along with protein-energy deficiency (PEM), iron, and vitamin A. Iodine deficiency has been shown to be a major factor in social and economic development (Stanbury, 1993; Bateman, 2004). Severe iodine deficiency results in Cretinism and goiter, and affects cognition, neuromotor capability, and brain function. Populations deficient in iodine are lethargic, thought to be lazy and non-responsive, and exhibit low IQs. In recent years spot populations in various parts of Europe and the U.S. have been found to have a high incidence of iodine deficiency.

The missing minerals ... iron, zinc, potassium, manganese, magnesium, and others

While cow's milk is rich in calcium and phosphorous, it does not fare so well in respect to several other minerals. An eight-ounce glass of milk, for example, provides only 1.5% of our daily requirement of iron, only 4.8% of our needed zinc, 4.4% of potassium, and 1.4% of our manganese. It notably lacks in another major mineral needed for bone maintenance, namely magnesium ... one glass supplying only 4.14% of our requirement. The low content of magnesium in milk is a much over-looked fact, which may explain part of the story why heavy milk-drinking populations still have high rates of osteoporosis. The ratio of recommended magnesium intake to calcium is 379 mg of magnesium to 1000 mg of calcium. But 4 glasses of milk, while providing 1,000 mg of calcium (100% of the RDA), only gives 90.8 mg of magnesium (24% of the RDA). Many feel that even this guideline ratio is too low ... some have suggested that a 2:1 ratio is more correct ... others have claimed even higher ratios yet, claiming that the role of magnesium has been grossly underestimated. Regardless, it is clear that milk does not provide sufficient amounts of magnesium to balance the calcium content.

Calcium, magnesium, and one other mineral, potassium, are also known to act as alkaline buffers in the body's acid-base balance homeostasis function. The low amounts of magnesium and potassium in milk contribute to milk and milk products' acid-producing property ... for example, cheeses have the highest 'potential acid renal load' (PARL) of all foods.

Other minerals supplied in low amounts in milk, compared to our RDA requirements, are copper and selenium ... although dairy industry advertisements often suggest that milk is an important source of both minerals, selenium in particular. In addition, the USDA Food Composition data base does not list the available amounts in milk for chloride, sulphur, arsenic, boron, chromium, floride, molydenum, nickel, silicon, and vanadium, so how milk fares in respect to these essential minerals is unknown. We do know from other sources, however, that cow's milk contains almost no boron or silicon, two minerals that are also noted to be essential to bone maintenance (Groff, 1995)

Fatty acids ... omega-3 ??

Another nutrient of concern is the essential fatty acid, linolenic acid, or 'omega-3'. We knew little of this substance, and the need for it, until we discovered that the Greenland Eskimos, who had copious amounts in their food supply, had no atherosclerosis or heart disease ... but could easily die from a simple nose bleed. We now know that this fatty acid, and the EPA and DHA that are the end products of its metabolic pathway, are critical for the maintenance of optimal health, especially in turning our metabolism away from excessive coagulation and inflammation ... and such things as the formation of plaque in our arteries. Further, we now know that the metabolic pathway of the second essential fatty acid, linoleic acid, or 'omega 6' leads to araachadonic acid and an opposing metabolic pathway favoring an inflammation and coagulation response. We also know that there is no homeostatic, or 'automatic' function by our physiologies to regulate which of these two pathways is prioritized ... the end production of araachadonic acid versus EPA and DHA depends solely on the amounts of each essential fatty acid we ingest, whether it is omega-3 or omega-6, and the successful completion of their two separate pathways.

It is theorized that once-upon-a-time in our humanoid ancestry we must have spent a long time in an environment that was rich in both linoleic and linolenic essential fatty acids, and thus lost, or never developed, a homeostatic function to regulate their pathways. This could have been a jungle environment, full of a large variety of plants, or maybe even near an ocean or large

18

lake. The lake area in East Africa could have been this environment. Regardless, it remains that we don't have a homeostatic function for these pathways, and so we are at the mercy of our own food choices and the amounts consumed.

We find, however, that we can 'cheat' if we ingest the EPA or DHA direct, as it is found in fish oil. However, we usually consume much more omega-6 in our diets, especially since the vastly increased consumption of vegetable oils in the form of margarines and cooking oils since we decided to drop using butter in favor of vegetable-based products after WWII. In addition, the availability of omega-3 has greatly diminished in more modern times. Wild grains and plants *do* contain substantial amounts of linolenic acid, as does the flesh of animals that feed on these wild plants. But linolenic acid is almost non-existent in domesticated grains and plants, and therefore the meat of animals that feed on these domesticated plants is also void of linolenic acid. As a result, there are very few good sources of omega-3 in our modern food supply. Among the common vegetable oils only the oil of the rapeseed, or 'canola' oil, and soybean oil, has any appreciable amounts. Flaxseed also has some … as does the oil from black walmuts. For any substantial amount of omega-3, however, we must therefore look to the end products of the pathway, EPA and DHA, found in ample supply in the fatty oils of fish such as salmon, cod, shrimp, tuna, mackerel, herring, and the King crab. In addition, the linolenic pathway is much more vulnerable to interruption than the linoleic pathway … by anti-oxidants, for example. It has been reported that an anti-oxidant presence equivalent to a daily intake of 250 mg of vitamin E will block the pathway.

There is also a major controversy about what *ratio* of omega-6 to omega-3 will optimize the health effect. Our current guidelines suggest a ratio of 13:1. There is considerable evidence to indicate that this ratio is greatly in error. S.B. Eaton and Melvin Konner, in their landmark studies of our ancestral

19

diets, find that the ratio in the diet of early man was very close to unity (1:1), and suggests that our physiologies are designed for that kind of ratio.

Much has been written about the value of milk in providing linoleic and linolenic acid. Cow's milk does have some amounts of these two essential fats, largely depending on the particular cow's feed. As noted, domesticated feed grains are lacking in linolenic acid, and so very little omega-3 ends up in the cow's milk. However, the USDA food composition data base indicates that an eight-ounce glass of whole milk will contain 0.27 grams of linoleic fat and 0.17 grams of linolenic fat. In lowfat milk the linoleic amount drops to 0.06 grams and the linolenic falls to 0.009 grams, which is because these two essential fatty acids are contained in the fat part of whole milk.

Regardless, the claim that milk provides ample amounts of either linoleic acid or linolenic acid does not hold ground. The USDA food composition data indicates that an 8-ounce glass of whole milk contains only 2% of the daily recommended amount of 13.5 grams of linoleic acid, and 12.6% of the recommended intake of 1.35 grams of linolenic acid (omega-3), if the current NIH recommendations for the ratio of omega-6 to omega-3 intake is 13:1. If the recommended ratio of omega-6 to omega-3 were to follow Eaton and Konner's recommended 1:1, however, then that eight-ounce glass of milk would provide only 1.2% of our needed omega-3 essential fatty acid

The author's conclusion, then, is that cow's milk is a poor source for the much needed essential fatty acids, especially omega 3.

Protein

Milk, as stated in a previous section, is commonly thought to be an excellent source of high quality 'complete' protein. In fact, there is a current fad evidenced from sales at the local health food stores that milk protein is being prized as a top source of protein for body-builders and the health-minded. This is particularly true in the case of whey protein, argued to be a 'fast' metabolizing protein, especially useful in preventing muscle protein catabolism, and is considered to be 'complete'. However, does our scientific knowledge of protein metabolism and the make-up of protein in milk genuinely support this celebrity status?

A central concept in protein metabolism is the 'amino acid pool(s)', which contains amino acids of dietary origin plus those contributed by the breakdown of body tissues. These pools of amino acids (AAs) then become available to the vast array of cells in the body via the blood stream, each cell drawing from this circulating pool the specific amino acids needed to fabricate the proteins for which that cell is programmed to make.

It is critical that the cells have the complete array of amino acids available that it requires in order to fabricate the specific protein that it wants to make, at that particular moment. This is where the concept of 'complete' amino acids enters the picture … also the source of much discussion and debate. A common misunderstanding is that the time factor is not critical … that if a missing essential amino acid is not available at that precise moment it can be derived from body tissue or obtained from the food source at a later meal. However, the body is slow to catabolize amino acids from body tissue and is relatively reluctant to do so. And, common sense tells us that if an essential amino acid is not available in the individual's food supply for a long enough duration, then the body tissues will also be lacking in that particular amino acid … the eight (nine for infants) essential amino acids cannot be fabricated by our bodies. In addition, the timing can be very swift … if the cell does not have the needed amino acids at hand, the amino acids which it does have are stripped of their nitrogen heads … which are excreted as urea … and the tails are sent to the cell's Kreb Cycle to be utilized for energy. The timing is more in the realm of seconds and minutes rather than hours. This is why it is not true

21

that incomplete proteins digested at different meals will combine their amino acids to provide the complete arsenal of essential amino acids. It is also the reason why the persistant consumption of incomplete proteins ultimately leads to whole-body protein deficiency. In respect to cow's milk this is very important, because milk protein is actually quite low in at least two essential amino acids.

The notion that cow's milk protein may be limiting in one or more essential amino acids has been known for a long time, but only in recent years has this received enough attention to warrant serious scientific study ... study that has been mostly sponsored by the dairy industry, directed at attempts to correct any imbalance, with the end goal of increasing production and consumer marketability. Factors affecting the amino acid composition of bovine milk protein include (a) the breed of cow and individual genetic composition, (b) relative quantity of milk production for the individual cow, (c) the lactation period at the time of milking, (d) the growth rate of the cow at the time of milking, (e) the health of the cow's mammary functions, (f) the cow's digestive health, and (g) the quality of its food supply. Alterations in type of feed, addition of protein supplementation, and administering specific drugs are the most common artificial factors that can alter amino acid composition.

Under 'normal' conditions the two most limiting bovine milk amino acids are methionine and lysine, with methionine being the most noted. For example, methionine is also the most limiting amino acid in legume plant foods, and it is known that the combination of cow's milk and legumes does not provide a 'complete' protein source (Gropper, Smith, Groff, 2005). It is important that lysine is a second limiting AA, because lysine is limiting in many other food protein sources, such as rice, and because it is comparatively more vulnerable to destruction by heat and other factors. In my other writings I refer to lysine as 'the littlest amino acid'.

Other limiting amino acids have been identified as well. On a traditional diet of grass silage and barley the most limiting AA was found by Korthonen et al (2002) to be histidine. This is very significant for babies fed cow's milk exclusively, since histidine is an essential AA for infants. Meijer et al (1995) found that glutamine is another potentially limiting AA in the high yielding cow. Abu-Ghazaleh et al (2001) added phenylalanine as a potentially limiting amino acid.

The type of feed has a marked effect on the amino acid composition of the cow's milk, and on milk production. Huller and Brand (1993) confirmed that milk from naturally foraging cows increased milk fat but depressed milk yield and protein content, compared to grain and meal feeds. The predominant feeds for the modern dairy herd are grains complemented with soybean meal, corn meal, and fish meal. Abu-Ghazaleh et al compared the effect on bovine blood amino acids of feed diets consisting of soybean meal, fish meal, or both. They found that methionine, lysine, and phenylalanine were the most limiting AAs in all diets. Fish meal slightly improved the methionine status. Wu et al (1997) determined that methionine *or* lysine were limiting when soybean meal was the protein source, but lysine was the predominantly limiting AA when corn gluten meal or brewer's grains were the source. Applied protein supplement concentrate with methionine and lysine was found to increase milk production as well as the milk content of these two AAs. (Wang et al, 2010)

In studies such as the above mentioned Meijer et al study (1995) and Schwab et al (1992), it was also confirmed that the milk content of amino acids, including methionine, phenylalanine, glutamine, and glycine was affected by the stage of lactation of the cow at the time of milking.

In sum, it is clear that bovine milk protein is not truly 'complete', but instead is seriously limiting in at least two essential amino acids. Coupled with the knowledge that

23

combining incomplete proteins to make the complete arsenal available to body cells is time sensitive, the implication is that meal planning and estimations of complete protein intake need to be done carefully and with good information.

3. An emerging consensus among scientists and health care professionals that human breast milk is best for infants, and using cow's milk as a substitute should be discouraged.

Since the year 1971, when the practice of breastfeeding reached an all-time low in America, there has been a growing consensus in the medical profession that cow's milk should *not* be fed to infants. In 1984 the office of the U.S. Surgeon General initiated the landmark "Surgeon General's Workshop on Breastfeeding" which delineated six priority breastfeeding issues and organized numerous events and actions. Their motto, "to protect, promote, and support breastfeeding" was championed by many other agencies and organizations in following years.

The current policy statements of representatives of the professional health care community, such as the American Academy of Family Physicians (AAFP), the American Academy of Pediatrics (AAP), and the American Dietetic Association are consistent with the conclusion that human milk is best for human babies.

4. Awareness that recommendations to consume milk and dairy products is not politically correct, considering that most non-white ethnic groups are lactose intolerant, and evidence that calcium requirements for non-white ethnic groups may be different.

5. Vegetarians propose that we should not be eating animal-based foods for health reasons.

6. Animal rights groups argue that animals raised for food are abused and mis-treated, especially by big-

business enterprises, and that perhaps we shouldn't be eating the flesh of other animal species for food.

7. A resistance by some people to purchase non-organic foods, or products produced by unscrupulous and overly profit-orientated big business, with questionable quality and product composition.

8. Negative consumer reaction to the treatment of cow's with rBGH, anti-biotics, and other substances ... administered for the purpose of increasing milk production.

9. The knowledge that commercial milk can be contaminated with blood, pus, manure, and other undesirable matter.

10. A reaction towards labeling laws that do not ensure that we know what is in the milk and milk products we consume ... plus concerns about false advertising.

11. The awareness of a possible contradiction between high calcium intake from dairy products and osteoporosis.

12. Accumulating scientific evidence linking cow's milk to a number of disease conditions in humans.

There is therefore a strong challenge to the notion that milk is "nature's most perfect food", albeit perhaps a valuable one never-the-less. However, there remains one remaining argument why we should perhaps not drink milk, at least the variety that has been identified as "Type A1" cow's milk, and which can generate a peptide harmful to our health, named BCM-7.

The Devil In The Milk

In this chapter we have now come a full circle. I started with a brief introduction to the Type A1/ A2 milk issue and the BCM-7 peptide, and then introduced the *good* and the *bad* of cow's milk. Now we have come back to the *ugly* .... the seven-amino acid beta-casomorphin peptide fragment which commonly separates from the 209 amino-acid-chain that makes up the beta-casein portion of Type A1 cow's milk protein, dubbed by Dr Keith Woodford as the *devil in the milk.* This is a continuation of the approach presented in the precedent to this expose, entitled *MILK ... to drink, or not to drink ??*

The presentation of the evidence that leads to the conclusion that the BCM-7 peptide poses serious health risks ... the chronological sequence of scientific research and studies ... reads like a long unfolding saga. This is the subject of the next chapter.

References For Chapter One

Abu-Ghazaleh, A.A.; Schingoethe, D.J.; Hippen, A.R.; *Blood amino acids and milk composition from cows fed soybean meal, fish meal, or both,* Journal of Dairy Science, 2001, May; 84(5): 1174-81.

Atkins, P.J.; White Poison? The Social Consequences of Milk Consumption, 1850-1930, Social History of Medicine, 1992; 5(2): 207-227.

Bateman, B.G.; *Nutrition Intervention: A Potential Factor For Economic Growth and Development,* Master of Science thesis, Mahidol University, Thailand, 2004

Berton, P.; Barnard, N.D.; Mills, M.; *Racial bias in federal nutrition policy, Part I: The public health implications of variations in lactase persistence,* Journal of the National Medical Association, 1999, March; 91(3): 151-7.

Crittenden, R.G; Bennett, L.E.; *Cow's Milk Allergy: A Complex Disorder,* Journal of the American College of Nutrition, Vol. 24, No. 90006, S825-5915, 2005

DuPuis, E.M.; *Nature's Perfect Food,* New York University Press, 2002

Eaton, S.B.; Konner, M.J.; *Paleolithic Nutrition: A Consideration of Its Nature and Current Implications,* New England Journal of Medicine, 312 (1985): 283-89

Eaton, S.B.; Shostak, M.; Konner, M.; *The Paleolithic Prescription,* Harper & Row, Publishers, 1988

European Food Safety Authority (EFSA), *Review of the potential health impact of β-casomorphins and related peptides,* Report of the DATEX Working Group on β-casomorphins, January 29th, 2009. Available online via the EFSA website: www.efsa.europa.eu/

Gropper, S.S.; Smith, J.L.; Groff, J.L.; *Advanced Nutrition And Human Metabolism,* Wadsworth, 2005, pp 219.

Hullar, I.; Brand, A.; *Nutritional factors affecting milk quality, with special regard to milk protein: a review,* Acta Veterinaria Hungarica, 1993; 41(1-2): 11-32.

Kikuchi, Y.; Takebayashi, T.; Sasaki, S.; *Iodine concentration in current Japanese foods and beverages,* Nippon Eiseigaku Zasshi, 2008, July; 63(4): 724-34.

Korhonen, H.; Pihlanto, A.; *Bioactive peptides: Production and functionality,* International Dairy Journal, January 16, 2006, 945-960

Korthonen, M., Vanhatalo, A.; Huhlanen, P.; *Effect of protein source on amino acid supply, milk production, and metabolism of plasma nutrients in dairy cows fed grass silage,* Journal of Dairy Science, 2002, December; 85(12): 336-51

Meijer, G.A.; Van der Muelen, J.; Bakker, J.G.; Van der Koelen, C.J.; VanVuuren, A.M.; *Free amino acids in plasma and muscle of high yielding dairy cows in early lactation,* Journal of Dairy Science, 1995, May; 78(5): 1131-41.

Montgomery, M.R.; *A Cow's Life,* Walker & Company, 2004

Schwab, C.G.; Bozak, C.K.; Whitehouse, N.L.; Olson, V.M.; *Amino acid limitation and flow to the duodenum at four stages of lactation. 2. Extent of lysine limitation.* Journal of Dairy Science, 1992, December; 75(12):3503-16

Stanbury, J.B., editor; *The Damaged Brain of Iodine Deficiency,* Cognizant Communication Corporation, 1993. The reference in the text was to Chapter 16, entitled *Impact of Iodine Deficiency on Development of the Andean World,* by R. Fierro-Benitez, which outlined the socio-economic impact of iodine deficiency in developing populations.

University of Guelph, *Introduction to Dairy Science and Technology: Milk History, Consumption, Production, and Composition; 2010* www.foodsci.uoguelph.ca/dairyedu/intro

USDA: *United States Department of Agriculture, Nutrient Database for Standard Reference.* Food composition data is taken from this reference and compared with the dietary reference intakes listed in the *USDA DRI Tables: Dietary Guidance: Food and Nutrition Information Center.* It should be noted that the USDA Food Composition Data Base is *the* primary reference source for the nutrient content of food, and is used worldwide. It is an extensive data base, with its beginnings dating back to 1891, when the first food composition tables were published by W.O Atwater and C.D. Woods, who assayed the refuse, water, fat, protein, ash, and carbohydrate content of 200 different foods. The current data base contains data for more than 130 nutrients for 7,538 different foods, and is continually being expanded and updated. The data base is the reference for all of the nutrition soft-ware programs, such as Food Processor, the Nutritionist series, Nutri Genie, and Nutri Base, and for almost all scientific evaluations. Only a few years ago the data base provided information for only 9 vitamins and 9 minerals, but now includes all of the 14 essential vitamins and 10 minerals. Still lacking, however, is data for the essential minerals chloride, sulphur, boron, arsenic, chromium, floride, molybdenum, nicked, silicon, vanadium, and iodine.

The food composition data base can be accessed on the internet at http://www.ars.usda.gov/nutrientdata, and the dietary reference intakes at http://www.nal.usda.gov/fnic .

Calculations of the nutrient composition of milk was carried out using these two references and then extrapolating values for an eight-ounce serving (8 ounces = 28.35 X 8 = 227 grams). The mean adult intake references were used for daily recommended intakes.

Wade, N.; *Lactose Tolerance in East Africa Points to Recent Evolution,* The New York Times, December 11, 2006

Wang, C.; Liu, H.Y.; Wang, Y.M.; Yang, Z.Q.; Liu, J.X.; Wu, Y.M.; Yan, T.; Ye, H.W.; *Effects of dietary supplementation of methionine and lysine on milk production and nitrogen utilization in dairy cows,* Journal of Dairy Science, 2010, August, 93(8): 3661-70.

Woodford, K.; *Devil In The Milk,* Illness, Health, and the Politics of A1 and A2 Milk, First published in 2007 by Craig Potton Publishing, Nelson, New Zealand, with a North American edition published by Chelsea Green Publishing, White River Junction, Vermont, in 2009. ISBN 978-1-60358-102-8

Wu, Z.; Polan, C.E.; Fisher, R.J.; *Adequacy of amino acids in diets fed to lactating dairy cows.* Journal of Dairy Science, 1997, August; 80(8): 1713-21

Chapter Two

THE EVIDENCE

One of the fascinating characteristics of science is that the individual pieces of a bigger picture, or puzzle, are often slowly and painstakingly worked out, bit by bit, piece by piece, no one really understanding how they will finally come together until after the fact.

And that is how it was with the BCM-7 peptide story.

A Note To The Reader:

Understanding scientific literature and the specialized terminology which they use can be very frustrating without at least a basic understanding of the 'scientific method' and the nuances of the different types of studies and research. If you are interested in a brief overview of the subject pertinent to this expose', I encourage you, the reader, to review my section entitled *An Intro to the Scientific Method, Research-Study Design, and Statistics* in the Appendix, section A,

What *IS* Type A1 and Type A2 Milk ?

Knowledge of the differences between breeds of dairy cattle and the characteristics of their milk go back to the time that humans first domesticated the lineage of the cow, beginning with the ancient *auroch*, or *Bos primigenius,* the giant primordial ox.

As reviewed in Chapter One, we now have about 920 different cattle breeds worldwide. Six breeds predominate in the United States and most Western countries, which are the Ayrshire, the Brown Swiss, the Guernsey, Jersey, Milking Shorthorn, and the Holstein-Friesian. The Holstein-Friesian, un-matched for its high production capability, originated from Germany, and is currently the predominant breed in the U.S., Europe, and other countries such as Canada, New Zealand and Australia. The milk produced by each of these many different breeds varies considerably in content, and, as stated in the previous chapter, the content can also be influenced by feed and local environmental factors.

The major protein in cow's milk is *casein*, which comprises 76 to 86% of the total milk protein, and is divided into alpha-casein, beta-casein, and gamma-casein, with alpha-casein being the major portion (60% of the total casein). Alpha-casein is further separated into 'alpha-s-casein' and 'k-casein'. The remaining 14 to 24% of the protein portion in milk is a variety of proteins collectively called 'whey proteins', of which *lactoglobulin* is the most common (7-12% of the total whey proteins). For our discussion of the BCM-7 molecule, however, the genetic differences in the beta-casein portion is where we draw attention to.

Genetic variations of β-casein protein in cow's milk

Of the casein protein portion, approximately 27% is 'beta-casein', with as many as 15 different variations found among the milks produced by the world's dairy cattle population, with the variations dependent on the separate cattle species and breeds. All beta-casein from all cow breeds, however, is comprised of a folded chain of 209 individual amino acids. Genetically, and historically, the original beta-casein amino acid sequence in cow's milk contained a 'proline' at position number 67. But the first sequence discovered via modern scientific investigation

31

found a 'histidine' at that position, and thus this variation was named A1. We now know that the original variation contained a 'proline' amino acid at position 67, but this version has never-the-less been dubbed the A2 variant. The switch to a histidine at position 67 is thought to be due to a mutation which occurred among one single breed or species a few thousand years ago ...which we now know is the Holstein/Friesian breed originating from Central Europe.

In my research of early scientific knowledge about the genetic variations in cow's milk, and in particular about variations in the casein protein, I found that scientific investigation into the variations goes back to at least 1961, with a study by R. Aschaffenburg entitled *Inherited casein variants in cow's milk.* In 1963 the same researcher published *Inherited casein variants in cow's milk. II. Breed differences in the occurrence of β-casein variants,* and in 1965 *Variants of milk proteins and their pattern of inheritance.* During 1964, a study by Thompson et al entitled *Genetic polymorphism in caseins of cow's milk. II. Confirmation of the genetic control of beta-casein variations* confirmed Aschaffenburg's earlier work. Six variations of the beta-casein in cow's milk were isolated, and were initially categorized as A, B, C, D, E, and F, reflecting the order in which they were identified.

An excellent 19-page review of the discoveries of the many variations of milk proteins in all the sub-species of *Bos genus* is presented by Formaggioni et al in their 1999 paper entitled *Milk Protein Polymorphism: Detection and Diffusion of the Genetic Variants in Bos Genus.* In their review they credit Aschaffenburg with identifying and naming the 'A' variety of β-casein with his 1961 and 1963 studies, and then credits Peterson et al and Kiddy et al with first identifying a change of the amino acid at position 67 of the β-casein, from Proline to Histidine, and a change from histidine to glycine at position 106. The A type β-casein was thus separated into A1 (with the histidine at position 67), A2 (with proline at position 67), and A3 (with glycine at position 106 instead of histidine). Their work was published in 1966.

In Table 3 of Formaggioni et al's paper, it shows that the change of position 67 from a proline to a histidine also occurs in other varieties of β-casein, and identifies the research that led to each of the findings. Although Aschaffenburg was not aware of the differences in 'A' β-casein that would lead to the separation into A1, A2, and A3, he *had* discovered that β-casein 'B' and 'C' also had the histidine at position 67, which he discovered at the same time that he isolated β-casein 'A'. However, with 'B' β-casein there was also a switch from serine to arginine at position 122. With 'C' β-casein there was also a switch from glucine to lysine at position 37, and a switch from serine P to serine at position 35.

Then, some 17 years later, two more β-casein variants were added … 'G' and 'H', and it was further discovered that the 'H' variant also had the histidine instead of a proline at position 67 … discovered by Han et al in 1983 and confirmed by Chung et al in 1995, and again by Han et al in 1996. Visser et al found that the 'F' β-casein also had the same change (1991 and 1995); and Chin & Ng-Kwai-Hang found that variant 'G' again had the histidine at position 67 (1997) … their work was confirmed by Dong & Ng-Kwai-Hang in 1998.

It was recognized from these studies that the most significant occurrence of the histidine instead of a proline at position 67 lay with the A1 β-casein, which accounts for the greater part of modern milk production. Never-the-less, the case of 'B' β-casein may be an interesting secondary concern, because the 'B' β-casein is relatively common in some parts of Europe.

Other researchers followed suit confirming the early work with A1, A2, and A3 variants by Aschaffenburg, Peterson & Kopfler, and Kiddy. By 1984 many other scientists and researchers were well versed with the concept of the A1 and A2 variations of beta-casein protein in milk, and understood that these variations were dependent on genetics. An example is the 1984 study by Ng-Kwai-Hang et al, entitled *Association of genetic variants of casein and milk serum proteins with milk, fat, and protein production by dairy cattle.* Ng-Kwai-Hang and his research team are noted for their additional work in this field. For example, one of their contributions is Chapter 16 of the well-known textbook *Advanced Dairy Chemistry* (2002). The chapter is entitled *Genetic polymorphism of milk protein,* which provides an authoritative 78-page overview of the genetic variants in milk proteins and the history of their discovery.

In summation, then, *Type A1* cow's milk is the term applied to all variations of cow's milk that contains a histidine amino acid at position 67 in the 209 AA chain of its casein protein, while Type A2 cow's milk refers to all milk variations that contain a *proline* amino acid at that same number 67 position.

What Are Peptides ?

With digestion of beta-casein in the human stomach and small intestine, the protein chain is first broken down into fragments, or short segments, which are called *peptides.* With the 209 amino acid sequence, the break-down into separate fragments can potentially create a large number of possible individual peptides. Several digestive enzymes act to facilitate the separation, such as 'pepsin', 'leucine amino peptidase' and 'pancreatic elactase'. However, the relative ease at which the chain breaks, and its location, depends on the structural characteristics of the individual amino acids. For example, a proline tends to stabilize a segment and holds the chain together, while a histidine causes the chain to bend where it joins with the previous amino acid, and allows the chain to separate at that location relatively easily. Several prolines close together tend to make that section exceptionally stable and resistant to further fragmentation. One important example is again the proline or histidine at position number 67.

Peptides can be biologically active

Many of the peptides are characterized by being 'biologically active', which means that they can have a biological effect on physiological processes within the human body. As mentioned in the previous chapter, a number of these peptides are known to play beneficial and protective roles. An example is with the position 57 through 66 segment. With the proline at position 67 the chain will sometimes separate in that area of the chain to form three specific peptides which are noted for their beneficial effect: (a) the ten amino acid peptide from position 57 through 66 which is known to inhibit one enzyme that is linked to aggravating neurological disorders, (b) the six amino acid peptide containing positions 59 through 64, which is known to lower blood pressure, and (c), the five amino acid peptide containing positions 59 through 63, which demonstrates a role in enhancing the body's immune response. However, with a switch from the proline to a histidine at position 67 these three peptides are prevented from separating ... instead the usual peptides separated are a seven-amino acid fragment containing positions 60 through 66, and a truncated form of this same peptide containing positions 60 through 64. The amino acid sequence in the seven-long chain is Tyrosine-Proline-Phenylalanine-Proline-Glycine-Proline-Isoleucine. It is also important to note that the last 4 amino acids in this sequence, numbers 60-66, are Proline-Glysine-Proline-Isoleucine. This will be discussed below.

As discussed, some peptides can exhibit a beneficial effect on human physiologies. On the other hand, some peptides can be downright *devilish*. For example, it was suspected for a very long time that something in cow's milk was the cause of certain ill health conditions in humans. One condition was identified as *cow's milk allergy*, and concern for this illness helped prompt

35

the movement to promote breast-feeding, beginning in the 1960s. Even during that decade it was recognized that the problem lay with the protein in milk, possibly with peptides from the casein portion. During the 89s and 90s a number of studies investigated which casein peptide could possibly be the connection to 'cow;s milk allergy'. Several peptides were targeted as the potential *devil*. One peptide was the 17 amino-acid chain 'bovine serum albumin peptide (ABBOS), first identified by Karjalainen et al in 1993. This peptide is still being much studied.

The β- casomorphins, and BCM-7

"Caso" meaning "like" and "morphin", short for "morphine". In 1979 Henschen et al (H. Teschemacher was the team leader), published a paper entitled *Novel opioid peptides derived from casein (beta-casomorphins). II. Structure of active components from bovine peptone.* This was the first finding that some casein peptide fragments were 'casein-casomorphins' … in other words, were opioid-active peptide fragments. These peptides, therefore, had opiate properties similar to that of the narcotics opium and morphine. One of the casomorphins identified in the Teschemacher study was the 'beta-casomorphin-7' peptide, the peptide fragment containing positions 60 through 66. "Beta-casomorphin-7" was eventually abbreviated to BCM-7 (although just when I couldn't determine) … and yes, *this is the BCM-7 peptide ... the devil in the milk !!* Teschemacher concluded in this 1979 study that these casomorphins were highly bioactive and may be associated with promoting disease conditions in humans.

The opiate-like beta-casomorphins all contain anywhere from 4 to 11 amino acids in their chain, and all start with tyrosine followed by a proline, and have another tyrosine or a phenylalanine in the third or fourth position. This is known to be an important structural form which fits or matches the binding sites of opioid receptors in the human body. With this structure the peptide can attach to receptors in the body that then enable opiate-related activity. It is noted that the removal of the tyrosine completely inhibits bioactivity.

The BCM-7 casomorphin is exceptionally potent. For example, it takes ten times the amount of the drug 'naloxone', which is used to counter the effects of morphine overdose, to counteract an equivalent amount of BCM-7. A five amino acid truncated form of beta casomorphin-7, dubbed BCM-5, exhibits an even stronger opiate effect. The drug naloxone is often used in studies to test the presence of BCM-7 or BCM-5 and their opiate effect.

BCM-7 and Type A1, A2 Milk

We can now pull the knowledge of A1 and A2 milk together with what we know about the BCM-7 peptide. We know that the seven amino acid chain (the BCM-7 segment) is highly unlikely to separate intact if the amino acid at position 67 is a proline, as in the A2 genetic variant … the original variant for *Bos taurus*. However, when this position is occupied by the amino acid histine, the chain folds at that point and the fragment 60 through 66 easily separates … and position 67 is a histine in the A1, B, C, F, G, and H casein variants.

It is important to note that not all beta-casomorphins have the same disruptive potential as bovince BCM-7. Kaminski et al (2007) lists six beta-casomorphins naturally occurring in bovine milk plus two in human milk. Yes, human milk also has beta-casomorphins … BCM-7 and BCM-8. The main difference is that the second proline position in bovine BCM-7 is instead a valine in human BCM-7, and the amino acid after the end isoleucine is a proline in human milk instead of a histidine. Thus human BCM-7 acts like an A2 peptide rather than an A1 peptide, and the opioid effect is greatly reduced.

How does BCM-7 from A1 beta-casein enter the body?

The BCM-7 peptide fragment derived from Type A1 beta-casein is broken off from the 209 amino acid chain during normal digestion in the human stomach and small intestine. It is a relatively large molecule, however, and has been thought to be too large to normally pass through the membranes of the small intestine wall. This is a highly debated factor giving support to the argument that the BCM-7 molecule cannot and does not present a health issue … simply because it does not enter the blood stream with normal digestion. This also *may* help to explain why the effects of the BCM-7 molecule have remained hidden from scientific investigation for so long. Or, the conclusion may be invalid … it may be that the BCM-7 molecule can, in fact, pass through the intestinal membrane, even during normal digestion.

This is still a controversial issue … there are a few studies that suggest that the BCM-7 molecule *can* pass through the small intestine lining even under normal digestion conditions. For example, Iwan et al (2008), in their study entitled *Transport of micro-opioid receptor agonists and antagonist peptides across Caco-2 monolayer,* investigated whether beta-casomorphins could pass through one specific area of the small intestine membrane, named Caco-2. They found that they could, indeed, pass through. The BCM-7 beta-casomorphin was one of the peptides tested.

Sienkiewicz-Szlapka et al confirmed the results of the Iwan et al study in their very recent publication entitled *Transport of bovine milk-derived opioid peptides across a Caco-2 monolayer* (April, 2009), published in the International Dairy Journal.

It is also known that the enzyme 'dipeptidyl peptidase 4' (DPP4), located on the intestine mesenteric tissue, can act to degrade the BCM-7 molecule and break it down into smaller

38

segments, such as the even stronger opioid BCM-5, which can pass through the intestinal lining more easily.

Several recent studies by various dairy scientists of a number of beneficial peptides with sequences up to twenty amino acids conclude that these peptides can also enter the blood stream intact with normal digestion, which again suggests that the seven-amino acid chain of the BCM-7 peptide is not too large to pass through the intestinal wall.

In addition, we know that the BCM-7 molecule can easily enter the blood stream if any of a variety of special conditions exist. The most important of these special conditions is one that is normal with infants … the digestive system of the newborn human baby is not fully developed and remains permeable to the transport of large molecules across the small intestine wall for at least the first six months, and often into early childhood. This means that *the BCM-7 molecule readily transfers into the blood stream of human babies.*

Further, persons may have what is termed a 'leaky gut' for a number of reasons and conditions, and this will also allow the BCM-7 molecule to enter the blood stream. These conditions include Celiac disease, ulcerative colitis, Crohn's disease, and stomach ulcers. It is interesting to note that a common treatment of stomach ulcers has been to drink milk … one example is the 'Sippy' high milk diet, which has also been related to an increased incidence of deaths due to heart disease. It is also worthy of mention that it has been found that individuals suffering from various neurological disorders, such as autism and schizophrenia, often have unusually permeable digestive systems, although this claim has been contested.

As mentioned in the first chapter, another factor which may play an important role in the ability of the BCM-7 peptide to enter the blood stream is the extended time duration that milk normally takes to digest … the milk 'mass' that enters the stomach after drinking a glass tends to linger longer than other food substances.

Diabetes and the BCM-7 Connection

Autoimmune response and IDDM

The possible association of the BCM-7 molecule with diabetes refers to 'insulin-dependent diabetes mellitus', or IDDM. This form of diabetes is more commonly called Type 1 diabetes, or juvenile-onset diabetes.

Other forms of diabetes include Type 2 diabetes, or 'late-onset diabetes', and 'gestational diabetes' (GDM), which is a form of carbohydrate intolerance. Both of these two other forms can be treated through dietary changes and health care.

The incidence of Type 1 diabetes accounts for 10-15% of the total incidence of all of the forms of the disease. It can appear at any age, although most commonly with infants, children, and juveniles. People with Type 1 diabetes must inject themselves with insulin several times a day and must follow a careful diet and exercise plan.

An autoimmune response refers to the action by the body's immune system to isolate and attack invading substances. More specifically, antibodies, or 'T-cells', are produced by the body's immune system to attack 'antigens', or foreign viruses, bacteria, or other harmful compounds. The presence of an antigen stimulates the immune system to produce these antibodies, which then attack the antigens, inactivating them, and help to remove them from the body. While antigens can be from pathogenic (diseases-causing) infections and viruses, they can also be organic molecules from internal or environmental sources. One molecule that readily prompts an autoimmune response is the BCM-7 peptide. Once the immune system has created an antibody for an antigen whose attack it has survived, it continues to produce antibodies to protect from further attacks by that same antigen.

Diabetes is a disorder of metabolism which interferes with the way the body uses digested food for growth and energy. A major part of the food we eat is broken down to synthesize glucose, the form of sugar in the blood. Glucose is then the main sources of fuel for the body. Once in the blood stream, glucose is distributed to the various cells for uptake. A hormone produced by the pancreas, *insulin*, is required to be present to initiate and control the uptake of glucose by the individual cells. The pancreas is a large gland positioned behind the stomach, and it is the *beta-cells* in the pancreas that produce the needed insulin. After food digestion the right amount of insulin to move glucose from the blood into the cells is secreted. In people with insulin-dependent diabetes mellitus, however, the beta-cells malfunction, or don't function at all, and either too little or no insulin is generated. Uptake of glucose into the cells is thus diminished, and glucose levels in the blood rise. As a consequence glucose spills into the urine and is excreted from the body. In this situation the body loses its main source of fuel and energy … even though the blood contains large amounts of glucose ... and a disease condition results. IDDM becomes clinically symptomatic when approximately 80 – 85% of the pancreatic beta-cells are destroyed, requiring insulin injection as an intervention measure.

Classical symptoms of IDDM, or Type 1 diabetes include increased hunger and frequent urination. Prolonged high glucose levels causes 'glucose absorption' and effects such as a change in vision due to excess glucose altering the shape of the eye lenses. A number of skin rashes can occur with diabetes, collectively known as 'diabetic dermadr'. A form of 'ketoacidosis' is also common, characterized by the smell of acetone. Rapid, deep breathing, nausea, vomiting, and an altered state of consciousness can be additional symptoms. Diabetics

41

often experience wound-healing problems, and swelling of the extremities. Amputation of arms or legs can be an extreme consequence, and even death.

The concept that insulin-dependent diabetes mellitus could be caused by the destruction of pancreatic beta-cells by an autoimmune response is also not new. The 81-page PhD dissertation by Paula Klemetti (1999) gives an excellent review of the literature and studies in that field up to that time, and tells us that W. Gepts in his study entitled *Pathologic anatomy of the pancreas in juvenile diabetes mellitus*, was the first to identify the role of autoimmune mechanisms in the destruction of the pancreatic beta-cells, leading to IDDM. That was in the year 1965. During the 70s, 80s, and 90s a large number of studies were conducted which addressed the autoimmune link with diabetes.

The consensus in the scientific community now concludes that Type 1 diabetes is characterized by the destruction of the insulin-producing beta cells in the pancreas by the body's own immune system. The immune system reaction which causes the beta cells to be attacked is known to be triggered by a number of possible factors, including genetic, disease, and environmental factors. The environmental factors, in turn, can include viruses, and diet. Suggested dietary factors, to take this one more step, have included wheat gluten and various milk proteins. Yes, milk proteins … which potentially could be whey protein or casein protein.

One must therefore appreciate that IDDM is a multi-factorial disease condition, and although the immune response mechanism has been isolated as the central probable cause, the trigger to the initiation of this mechanism could be the result of any of a number of factors … which include milk protein.

Bringing the pieces of the puzzle together

By sometime in the early 1980s two separate pieces of our puzzle were therefore apparent, but had not yet been connected. It was known that (1) there were differences in the make-up of the casein protein in milk and that strongly bioactive peptides could be generated which prompted an autoimmune response, and (2) that the mechanism leading to insulin-dependent diabetes mellitus was probably the destruction of the pancreas beta-cells by an autoimmune attack. But putting the two concepts together had not been done.

How the auto-immune attack was triggered was therefore a central question at the time. One clue that pointed in the direction of milk protein presented itself during this period, however, and that was the fact that infants and young children with IDDM frequently and consistently had residues of milk protein antigens and the corresponding antibodies within their blood stream. The presence of specific milk protein antigens and their matching antibodies in infants with IDDM strongly suggested a causal link between the consumption of milk protein and the onset of IDDM in infants. These studies were used during those earlier years as support for the promotion of breastfeeding, and also to encourage manufacturers of commercial infant formulas to process the milk proteins to render them less reactive biologically. One such process was a technique to *hydrolyze* the milk protein. At the time the main concern was *cow's milk allergy*. It was thought that only infants with certain conditions which led to high risk were susceptible. Investigators did not, however, associate the allergy condition with any specific milk variety, although milk caseins were then suspected to be a likely source.

Robert Elliott

Robert Elliot and Martin, in their 1984 study *Dietary proteins: a trigger of insulin-dependent diabetes in the BB rat?* were the first to find evidence that the antigen prompting the autoimmune mechanism that Gepts had identified back in 1965 was a response to protein contained in cow's milk (at that time termed 'CM proteins').

Professor Bob Elliott was a diabetes researcher at Auckland University in New Zealand and was working mostly with animal models, particularly the BB rat, which is a rat breed known to be especially susceptible to the onset of diabetes. With his beginning studies Elliott knew that milk protein was strongly linked with promoting diabetes in the BB rat, but it was not clear which protein was the culprit, nor was Elliott aware of the different genetic variants in the milk proteins, particularly casein.

Additional studies investigating the relationship between milk proteins and IDDM

During the late 1980s and 90s a number of studies continued to investigate the connection of milk protein with human autoimmune reactions and disease risk, particularly IDDM. The Glarum et al study in 1989 was one of the first to propose that antigens to bovine milk protein could be the initiating factor in the onset of IDDM. Another study was by Dahl-Jergensen et al (1991). Fava et al published a study in 1994 entitled *Relationship between dairy product consumption and incidence of IDDM in childhood in Italy.* In 1997 W. Karges and his group confirmed that T-cell response to both pancreatic beta-cell antigens and milk proteins demonstrated mimicry … in other words, the autoimmune response to beta-cell antigens and milk proteins were identical, or at least very similar Further examples were a number of studies generated by the Childhood Diabetes in Finland Study (Virtanen et al, 1998, 2000).

More recently, Mikael Knip and his study group tested the relationship between the onset of IDDM in childhood with regular cow's milk versus highly hydrolyzed cow's milk, and concluded:

"Our data suggest that weaning to a highly hydrolyzed formula, as compared with a cow's-milk-based formula, was associated with a decreased risk of positivity for at least one diabetes-associated autoantibody ..." (Knip, 2010)

An interesting part of this study was the use of 'hydrolyzed' milk, which is a technique used to deactivate biological activity of protein peptides. More about this later.

Several milk proteins were thought to be the potential cause of the antigens, and different mechanisms were hypothesized. One of the protein peptides investigated was the 17 amino-acid chain 'bovine serum albumin peptide (ABBOS), first identified by Karjalainen et al in 1993. But none of these studies had yet targeted the 7-amino acid segment in β-casein at positions 60 through 66 ... the BCM-7 peptide.

Back to Robert Elliott

Keith Woodford reports in his book, *Devil In The* Milk, that sometime in 1993 Professor Robert Elliott telephoned the New Zealand Dairy Research Institute (NZDRI), asking to speak to someone who knew about cows and milk-protein biochemistry. Dr. Jeremy Hill took the call. The question was: is there a significant chemical difference in the proteins of milk from different cows ?? Hill then clarified that, yes, there is indeed a difference, which can separate the milk into two broad categories: A1 milk and A2 milk. Elliott then compared the incidence of IDDM with his mice, feeding them A1 and A2 milk. In his preliminary study, all the mice fed A1 milk developed IDDM and died. None of the mice fed A2 milk became diabetic.

It is interesting to note that the A1 and A2 milk samples used by Elliott in his work with mice was supplied by the New Zealand Dairy Research Institute, with funding from the New Zealand Dairy Board. In addition, Jeremy Hill, from NZDRI, was a co-researcher in some of those early studies.

One of Elliot's population studies during that same period compared Samoan children living in New Zealand with children living in their native homeland. Children in Samoa at the time consumed almost no milk, but Samoan children living in New Zealand did ... a lot ... like other New Zealanders. He found a ten-fold difference in the incidence of diabetes between the two children groups.

But he also knew that the incidence of diabetes varies greatly between countries ... as much as by a factor of more than 300 ... and that the variation could not be explained by *total* milk consumption alone. Finland, for example, consumes the highest amount of cow's milk and has the highest incidence of diabetes. But the populations of nearby France and Iceland also consume high amounts of bovine milk, yet have much lower rates of diabetes. This is especially true with Iceland. He had also studied the Masai people of Kenya, who consumed very large quantities of cow's milk, yet had an almost zero incidence of type 1 diabetes.

With his new knowledge of the difference between A1 and A2 milk Robert Elliot was thus pointed in the direction of undertaking further epidemiological studies in human populations to specifically compare diabetes and other diseases with the consumption of these two different types of milk.

The Pozzilli study

In 1996 Cavallo et al (Pozzilli was their team leader) studied the beta-casein peptides, in particular the sequence 60-66 in the 209 amino-acid beta-casein chain. They made a remarkable discovery: the 4-amino-acid sequence at the end of the 7-amino acid fragment was the same as the number 415 – 419 residues of the pancreas beta-cell glucose transporter molecule, named GLUT-2. This amino acid sequence was Proline-Glysine-Proline-Isoleucine. This was mentioned in a previous section. Cavallo and Pozzilli were thus the first to recognize that this particular peptide fragment possessed special characteristics that made it a likely candidate for a role in an autoimmune reaction involving the pancreas beta-cells. They suggested that the antibodies attacking the cow's milk casein fragment with the 60 – 66 amino-acid sequence would inadvertently also attack the GLUT-2 molecule in the beta-cell, thus rendering the beta cell function inoperable.

Pozzillis' reputation as a scientist and a specialist in the field of diabetes is impeccable. The reference at the end of this chapter highlights some of his achievements. His work lent considerable credibility to the BCM-7 – GLUT-2 proposed mechanism.

Additional studies linking Type A1 milk and the BCM-7 peptide with IDDM

Besides peer reviews of published studies, scientists often share their findings and research data directly among fellow scientists and associates working in the same field, whom they become acquainted with by correspondence or at scientific symposiums and conferences. News of Elliott's work apparently spread, and generated interest and further studies in other parts of the gobe.. One example is a study by I. Thorsdottir and O. Reykdal of Iceland in 1997 entitled *Food and the low incidence of IDDM in Iceland.* Their conclusion was as follows:

47

"The incidence of IDDM is lower in Iceland than among the genetically related nations of Scandinavia. Recent animal research in New Zealand has pinpointed a specific protein fraction in cow's milk, A1 β-casein, as one of the possible causes of an immunological destruction of the pancreatic β-cells resulting in IDDM. Milk protein allele frequencies in the Nordic cattle breeds varies, and preliminary results indicate that A1 β-casein is especially low in Icelandic milk."

Thorsdottir then completed a second study entitled *Different β-caseub fractions in Icelandic versus Scandinavian cow's milk may influence diabetogenicity of cow's milk in infancy and explain low incidence of insulin-dependent diabetes mellitus in Iceland.* Jeremy Hill was listed as one of the seven authors, and the study was published in the journal Pediatrics in 2000. The conclusion to this study was:

"The lower fraction of A1 and B β-casein in Icelandic cow's milk may explain why there is a lower incidence of IDDM in Iceland than in Scandinavia."

A third study, again with Jeremy hill, was published in 2002 and was entitled *Variations in consumption of cow milk proteins and lower incidence of Type 1 diabetes in Iceland vs the other 4 Nordic countries.* The conclusion was:

"… A1 and B beta-casein may contribute to varying diabetolgenicity of cow's milk and explain the difference in incidence of Type 1 diabetes." (Birgisdottir et al, 2002)

Thorsdottir showed up once more as co-author of a study entitled *Lower consumption of cow milk protein A1 beta-casein at 2 years of age, rather than consumption among 11- to 14-year old adolescents, may explain the lower incidence of type 1 diabetes in Iceland than in Scandinavia*, and was published in the journal Annals of Nutrition and Metabolism, 2006

(Birgisdottir et al, 2006). The title of the study is also their conclusion. This conclusion makes sense, considering that infants exhibit a more permeable digestive system with allows the BCM-7 casomorphin peptide to enter the blood stream.

It should also be noted that Jeremy Hill was one of the total of four authors (once again). Hill was with Fonterra at the time of Thorsdittir's fourth study, and Fonterra was then engaged in all-out war with A2 Corporation and the entire A1/A2 (BCM-7) hypothesis … in other words, he was working for a company which at the time was taking a stance *against* the A1 milk and BCM-7 hypothesis.

Even more pertinent, Thorsdottir later became one of the authors of the 2009 EFSA Report. More about this in the next chapter.

Professor Robert Elliott returns

In 1999 Elliott and his research team completed and published a study entitled *Type 1 (insulin-dependent) diabetes mellitus and cow milk: casein variant consumption.* The study built on previous work comparing IDDM in 0 to 14-year-old children from 10 countries, using national annual cow milk protein consumption data. Their finding was that although total protein consumption did not correlate with the incidence of diabetes, consumption of the beta-casein A1 variant definitely did. The 'correlation coefficient was $r = 0.726$. Even more pronounced was the relation between beta-casein 'A1+B' consumption and IDDM, with a correlation coefficient of $r = 0.928$. As I stated in the previous paragraphs, the 'B' variant of β-casein can also produce the seven amino acid β-casein peptide fragment from positions 60 through 66 (BCM-7). Milk containing the B variant of β-casein was relatively common in the populations he targeted. The calculated degree of correlation is nothing short of astonishing.

It was not until 2003, however, that Elliot and his co-worker, Laugesen, were able to complete a larger between-country correlation study and finally draw a higher level of attention to their research. They compared mortality (death rate) due to ischaemic heart disease (HCD) and the incidence of Type 1 insulin-dependent diabetes mellitus (IDDM) with consumption of A1 and A2 milk in 20 countries. The correlations, similar to their previous study, were extremely high: for ischaemic heart disease and A1 cow milk proteins, 'r' equaled 0.92 (p < 0.00001); for Type 1 diabetes mellitus r equaled 0.76 (p < 0.001). These were amazingly high correlation values.

What does this measured correlation mean? A correlation of 1.0 indicates a one hundred percent equivalent incidence of the two factors being compared, which *suggests* that the one *causes* the other ... or is caused by the same factor. The measure of correlation is the 'correlation coefficient, 'r', and is a measure of the linear relationship between two variables. If the relationship between two variables is non-linear, meaning that the incidence of the one variable does not move consistently with changes in the other variable, then the r – value has no significance. In statistical analysis, a correlation of 0.76 is very high, and 0.92 is exceptionally high. However, we must always keep in mind that correlation does not prove causation.

Another statistical technique is to square the 'r' value to obtain the 'coefficient of determination' which tells us the percent of the data that is 'closest to the line of best fit'. An r^2 value of 0.85 means that 85% of the total variation between the two variables can be explained by the proposed association, and only 15% can possibly be explained by other factors. The 'r^2' values for the correlation of A1 milk with heart disease and diabetes in Elliott's and Laugessen's study was 0.58 and 0.85, respectively.

The p-values calculated by Laugesen and Elliott are also significant. The p-value is the probability of obtaining a test statistic at least as extreme as the one that was actually observed. A p–value of 0.001 (one in a thousand chance) is the accepted norm for a credible association, which is what was derived for the diabetes association. And p = 0.00001 (one in a one-hundred-thousand chance), derived for the heart disease association, is considered exceptional. The strength of association found in the 2003 Laugessen and Elliott study is remarkable, and if not refuted, is by itself reason to take notice. It must also be noted that Elliot and Laugesen explored possible confounders extensively, finding none that could effectively counter their conclusions. Their work has been criticized, yes, and confounders have been proposed … but the credibility of their work remains high … *very* high !!

Heart Disease and the BCM-7 Connection

Corran McLachlan

The saga continues … for the years 2000 through 2006 I rely heavily on Keith Woodford and his remarkable book, *Devil In The Milk*. During this period additional scientific study supporting the BCM-7 hypothesis was published, A2 Corportation was conceived and formed, Fonterra took over as the New Zealand dairy industry leader, and the 'great debate' emerged.

Corran McLachlan was a rare individual. As Woodford describes him, "He was one of those few people who could cross disciplines and make the great leaps needed to advance our understanding about the world we live in. He was also a man of great passion. But he was also a person who could work away painstakingly, putting together the detailed analyses on which the great leaps in knowledge are built." (pp 21) His achievements make a long list, and include 'Head Boy' and 'Senior Athletic Champion' at Wairarapa College, N.Z.; a first class honors degree in Chemical Engineering at Cambridge

University, England; was the recipient of the first United Development Corporation Inventor's Prize in 1974; was General Manager at New Investments; Executive Director of Duncan & Davies Nurseries Ltd., and finally Managing Director of Tenon Development Ltd. McLachlan authored 29 scientific papers and confidential reports and held 11 patents.

In the year 1994 Corran McLachlan was asked by the New Zealand Child Health Research Foundation to review Robert Elliott's research program. At that time McLachlan had been working on processes to manufacture low-cholesterol and cholesterol-free foods. McLachlan was struck by the similarity in Elliott's data and that which he had encountered in his own work … data concerning IDDM incidence rates, and death rates due to ischaemic heart disease. He became strongly convinced that Elliott was on the right track, and began his own research. The businessman part in him also urged him to seek out how this new evidence could be put to use to make money.

In 2001 he published a meta-analysis study in the journal Medical Hypotheses entitled *Beta-casein A1, ischaemic heart disease mortality, and other illnesses*. The study used data from the World Health Organization (WHO) MONICA project and compared the incidence of ischaemic heart disease with the consumption of type A1 milk.

The "Multinational Monitoring of Trends and Determinants in Cardiovascular Disease Project", known as the MONICA Project, was established in the early 1980s in a number of centers around the world to monitor trends in cardiovascular diseases, and to relate these to changes in risk factors in the populations over a ten year period. There were a total of 32 MONICA Collaborating Centers located in 21 countries. The total number of men and women monitored, aged 25-84 years of age, exceeded ten million. The results were tabulated and published in the late 1990s, and the data are still being used for analysis even today.

McLachlan calculated that the correlation between ischaemic heart disease mortality and the consumption of type A1 milk was $r = 0.927$, and $r^2 = 0.86$. This calculation was similar to that concluded in the 1999 study by Elliott et al, and again the study by Elliott and Laugesen in 2003.

McLachlan also compared the incidence among the specific populations of Toulouse, France and Belfast, Ireland. The MONICA data showed that these two populations were almost identical in collective risk factors traditionally identified for heart disease. However, the consumption of Type A1 milk in Belfast was 3.23 times that in Tolouse, *and* the heart disease mortality rate in Belfast was similarly just over three times that of Toulouse.

Including data about Type 1 diabetes, McLachlan was also able to show that the incidence of this disease closely matched with that of ischaemic heart disease in the populations studied, thus suggesting that the two disease conditions shared a common causative factor.

McLachlan also discussed the paradox of a very high consumption of cow's milk among the Masai and Samburu people of Kenya, who, surprisingly, have a very low incidence of heart disease ... it was known that the dairy cattle of these peoples produces only A2 milk. The Finland and French paradox was also revealed: The Fins are one of the highest per capita consumers of cow's milk in the world, and also with almost the highest incidence of heart disease ... the French consume a high per capita amount of cow's milk as well, yet their incidence of heart disease is much lower than in Finland. The milk consumed in Finland is from almost exclusively A1 cows, while the 'Normande' French breed produces close to pure A2. His observations and suggested conclusions were supported with statistics and graphical analysis.

An aside: some have picked up on the French paradox, noting that this offers yet another explanation as to why the French have a lower incidence of heart disease compared to other European populations. It was proposed some time ago that it was because the French consumed less saturated fat, and then later because of something in the grape seeds used to make French red wine ... it may be that both these explanations are incorrect ... that it is instead because French cows produce Type A2 milk?

In March, 2003, McLachlan published a letter in the New Zealand Medical Journal entitled *Setting the record straight: A1 β-casein, heart disease and diabetes*, which defended his 1999 study and went on to summarize additional statistical data demonstrating the strong epidemiological correlation between Type 1 diabetes and ischaemic heart disease mortality, emphasizing that a common factor was at play, and that this link could be the consumption of Type A1 milk.

Although McLachlan was recognized for authoring these two valuable publications, his main contribution regarding the A1/A2 hypothesis was his influence in conveying the relevant science and data to the N.Z. Dairy Board and the N.Z. Dairy Research Institute. McLachlan was convinced that A1 beta-casein, and the BCM-7 peptide derived from it, comprised a major public health issue.

In Feberuary, 2000, McLachlan joined with New Zealand entrepreneur Howard Paterson to form a company named A2 Corporation. The concept was to commercialize the marketing of A2 milk by way of franchising and forming agreements with milk processors and marketers. This included copyrighting 'A2 Milk' as A2 Corporation's own brand, and patenting procedures to test dairy herds and milk samples for A1 versus A2 properties. NZ$12.8 million in capital was raised in the first year, with McLachlan assuming the position of Chief Executive and owning 35% in return for his intellectual property.

The details of how this came to pass makes fascinating reading, and is part of Woodford's writing … well worth reading.

BCM-7 and oxidation of LDL ??

Given that an A1 milk/autoimmune mechanism may be at play with diabetes, and the observed close correlation between the incidence of Type 1 diabetes and ischaemic heart disease, then the question arises: "what, then, is the possible mechanism by which the devil in the milk can contribute to heart disease ??"

Ischaemic heart disease (IHD), or 'myocardial ischaemia' is a disease characterized by a reduced blood supply to the heart muscles, usually due to blockage in the arteries, such as by the formation of arterial 'plaque', or the build-up of fatty materials such as cholesterol. The resultant thickening of the arterial walls, also known as 'atherosclerosis' slows down or stops the passage of blood, leading to a 'starved' condition and cellular death in the affected muscles. In the case of the heart this causes failure of heart muscle function, or 'myocardial infarction' (heart attack).

Atherosclerosis is still not well understood, but there is a strong consensus that the oxidation of 'low-density-lipoprotein' (LDL) is a key factor. It may act via oxidized LDL to damage arterial walls and then to become part of the actual plaque build-up, or it may simply be the material used in the build-up. With either scenario, this is where BCM-7 enters the scene … BCM-7 is known to be a strong oxidant.

Once again there is a paucity of supportive studies, and there are a number of articles and studies which attempt to refute the premise that the BCM-7 peptide may be linked to LDL oxidation. Four supportive studies stand out: one by Torreilles et al in 1995, one by Tailford et al in 2003, and a pair of studies by Steinerova et al in 1999 and 2001. All four studies have been strongly criticized, and the Steinerova studies do not directly address the possible role of beta-casomorphins.

The study by the French scientist, Jean Torreilles, and his co-worker, Marie-Christian Guerin is by far the most directly supportive study. Titled *Casein-derived peptides can promote human LDL oxidation by a perosidase-dependent and metal-dependent process,* they were able to demonstrate under laboratory conditions that the 'tyrosyl radical' (a free radical, generated by damaged tyrosine amino acid) could act as a catalyst to oxidize LDL lipids. (Torrielles, 1995) Their work has been much discussed, but not refuted.

Tailford et al (Julie Campbell was the leader and corresponding author) took this a step further with their study in 2002, using rabbits as test animals. They were able to show that rabbits fed type A1 beta-casein developed fatty plaque lesions that were both larger and thicker than those of rabbits fed A2 beta-casein. Unfortunately, they were not able to demonstrate that the correlation was statistically significant, and the study was further criticized because it was commissioned by A2 Corporation.

Again there is a great need for high-quality, credible studies. Never-the-less, the Torreilles and Tailford studies, even by themselves, do give credible evidence that the BCM-7 peptide is a strong oxidant, and *does* have the capability to oxidize LDL cholesterol.

An aside: Vitamin C, the BCM-7 peptide, and infant atherosclerosis

At this point I would like to introduce a hypothesis of my own, the basis of which is suggested in the studies related in the previous sections.

Food composition studies (USDA) reveal that cow's milk contains virtually no vitamin C. It actually makes sense that it doesn't … the momma cow doesn't need vitamin C in her food supply because her body makes its own. And her baby calf doesn't need it in the mother's milk either … it makes its own as well. And, there is no or very little in the grass and grains the mother cow feeds on anyway.

But it is very important for us humans that we obtain vitamin C in our food, because we need it urgently, and *we do not manufacture our own, unlike almost all other animals.* We belong to a small select portion of the animal kingdom whose bodies does not produce their own vitamin C, which includes the gorilla, the chimpanzee, the guinea pig and the fruit bat, and one species of birds. We possess nearly all of the metabolic pathway to produce the vitamin, but lack the final enzyme needed to complete the pathway … the liver enzyme *gulonolactone-oxidase.* This suggests that at one time in our evolution, probably common with the gorilla and chimpanzee, we lived in an environment so rich in vitamin C that we didn't need to manufacture our own and therefore lost the ability to do so.

Vitamin C has a number of roles in our metabolism, the most noteworthy being an essential nutrient in the formation of 'collagen', the connective tissue which binds so many of our bodily components together, such as in our skin and our arteries. A deficiency in vitamin C results in the disease condition 'scurvy' in which blood vessels rupture, our gums lose their integrity and our teeth fall out, along with loss of hair, and the body begins to rot. The Scottish called the condition 'black legs' due to the formation of black patches under the surface of the skin caused by the rupture of blood capillaries. Before it was known that the consumption of citrus fruits could remedy the condition, sailors suffered terribly from scurvy … during sea battles and the age of exploration many more deaths were the result of scurvy than injury in battle. It was a serious problem among the Mormon pioneers when they crossed the great plains on the way to Utah, and even during WWI and WWII.

The lack of vitamin C in cow's milk can then be a serious shortcoming ... vitamin C is of course vital for the growth of prenatal and newborn babies, and throughout infancy. It may be lacking in human mother's milk as well, as the amount present in breast milk depends entirely on the mother's intake of the nutrient from her food. If she is lacking in vitamin C, so will her breast milk.

It has been known for a long time that advanced arterial plaque build-up, or atherosclerosis, can be evidenced in young adults, children, and even infants as young as 1 to 2 year olds. This startling phenomenon was first discovered during autopsies of soldiers during WWII, followed with further studies in children and infants. A credible explanation for this condition in humans so young has never gained any general consensus, and is the source of controversy to this day. However, I propose that the combination of a lack of vitamin C and the presence of the BCM-7 oxidant peptide may well be the fundamental cause.

Mainstream medical science has long stressed the role of oxidized LDL in the formation of arterial plaque, but little has been addressed to the question of *why* the body chooses to form plaque in the arteries in the first place ... although there is clear agreement in the medical literature and physiology textbooks that there was an starting 'incident' to prompt the beginning of the plague formation. What is meant by 'incident' is that the arterial wall was damaged or in a weakened condition. Very little investigation has been directed to this 'damage' or 'weakened condition'. One theory is that oxidized LDL itself causes damage to the arterial wall, and then secondly becomes the base material with which to form the plaque build-up. But a growing number of scientists now conclude that a weak or subnormal arterial wall structure is directly due to poor collagen formation caused by a lack of needed nutrients, most notably vitamin C.

Then, if an infant was fed on cow's milk, especially exclusively, the stage would be set for that infant to be lacking in vitamin C and to present deficient collagen in its arterial wall structure, and to prompt the formation of atherosclerosis. In this respect, it is interesting to note that, at least in the U.S., exclusive bottle-feeding with cow's milk was very common throughout the 20th century, with breast-feeding reaching its lowest rate of practice in 1971, and that most of the infant formulas, both home-made and commercially prepared, were based on cow's milk.

Then add to this the knowledge that the BCM-7 oxidative peptide can easily pass through the permeable intestinal walls of the infant. The infant's intestinal apparatus does not reach maturity until approximately 2 years of age. So we then have present in the cow's-milk-fed-infant not only a cause for weak arterial walls, but also a peptide in the main food source that readily oxidizes LDL and thus promotes its application in the formation of atherosclerosis.

One further piece of information that fits into the puzzle and helps form the bigger picture is that we also know that formation of atherosclerosis at a young age precludes the continued formation during following years … the condition does not seem to readily reverse or even to stabilize.

Now … this analogy is strictly mine, the author's. I know of no studies that specifically conclude this same theoretical explanation, although the individual pieces of the puzzle are substantiated by research and are credible. This is an example of the urgent need for more specific research and scientific study in nutrition-related causes of disease. The failure for such research to take place is a direct result of complacency by government agencies, the suppressive power of special-interest orientated industry, and a paradigm in medical science that accentuates the drug approach and ignores the importance of nutrition in our bodily function and health.

The Connection of the Opiate BCM-7 Peptide, and Neurological Disorders

The proposed link between autism, schizophrenia, and other neurological diseases with gluten (wheat protein) and casein (milk protein) has been around for a long time. The treatment of consuming a diet free of these two proteins … named the 'gluten-free, casein-free (GFCF) diet … has been tried by a large number of individuals over more than four decades, with a very long list of positive testimonials.

One of the first to connect autism and schizophrenia with diet was Dr. Curtis Dothan in the early 1960s. He identified a phenomenon that suggested the linkage, which was the observation that schizophrenic sufferers very often had unusually permeable digestive systems and digested both the gluten protein from wheat and the casein protein from milk 'inefficiently' … meaning that upon digestion the protein failed to break down completely into individual amino acids, but instead was characterized by the formation of peptide fragments. Dr. Jaak Panksepp reported the same observations in 1979.

The theory was given new insight when Dr. Kalle Reichelt found that gluten and casein peptides were commonly present in the urine of autistic children, but not in the urine of normal children. Reichelt supported Dothan's suggestion that upon digestion by autistic (and schizophrenic) sufferers, the proteins were not broken down completely into individual amino acids, but instead allowed some fragments, or peptides, to break away intact, and these peptides could then pass through abnormally permeable stomach or intestinal linings. This phenomenon is once again our 'leaky gut' scenario. However, it is important to note that in the autistic or schizophrenic what may be critical is the combination of inefficient digestion of the proteins on one hand, with a permeable, or 'leaky gut' on the other. The theorized passage of protein peptides and presence in the blood stream is a result of, first, incomplete digestion into individual amino acids, and secondly, the ability of the larger peptide fragments to pass through a leaky gut.

Now, this can explain how a peptide or beta-casomorphin may enter the body. However, if the peptide is causally associated with neurological dysfunction, they must be able to enter the brain. But our designers gave us a marvelous gift to prevent damage to that most crucial part of our body ... the *blood-brain barrier*. Abbreviated BBB, the blood-brain barrier is a separation of circulating blood and cerebral fluid ... the fluid that our brain literally 'floats' in. The barrier occurs along all blood capillaries going to the brain and consists of tight junctions that are unique to only that area. 'Endothelial cells' restrict the passage of microscopic objects such as bacteria and larger 'hydrophilic' molecules (are non-soluble in water), yet allow 'hydrophobic' (water-soluble) molecules to pass. These hydrophobic molecules include hormones and oxygen. Certain cells of the barrier also actively transport minerals, glucose, and other compounds via specific barrier proteins.

So ... the question is then asked: "Can the opioid peptides such as BCM-7 (and gliadorphin) cross the blood-brain barrier? In 1999 Drs Robert Cade and Zhongjie Sun et al completed a study with rats that demonstrated conclusively that yes, the BCM-7 beta-casomorphin can pass through the blood-brain barrier. (Sun et al, 1999).

Thus one more piece to the puzzle was put in place.

It is also crucial to understand that the peptides from wheat gluten can be very similar to those derived from casein. I was surprised in my research to find that much of what we now know about gluten peptides is relatively new knowledge.

Our cereal grains, as we now know them, are a relatively new food for us humans. Similar to the case of cow's milk, we did not domesticate cereal grains such as wheat until about 9,000 years ago ... perhaps 2,000 years before we domesticated *Bos*

61

taurus, the cow. This has been suggested to be one reason why we have trouble with cereal proteins ... our physiologies may simply not be designed for this come-along-lately food.

The nutritional value of the grains make them an important food choice, however. One hundred grams of hard red winter wheat, for example, contains about 71 grams of carbohydrate, 1.5 g of total fat, 12.2 g of dietary fiber, and 12.6 grams of protein, and is an important source for many vitamins and minerals, notably iron. The main protein is 'gluten' which comprises about 80% of the protein in wheat. It is also the main protein in rye and barley.

Gluten is the composite of two proteins, named *gliadin* and *glutenin*. It is important to note that, although the proteins in maize and rice are sometimes called gluten, they do not contain the gliadin portion. Gliadin, similar to casein, can separate into peptide fragments, and these peptides can also have opiate properties. The most significant is the seven amino acid chain called *gliadorphin,* or *gluteomorphin.* Yes ... a 7-amino acid fragment !! The amino-acid sequence is Tyr-Pro-Gly-Pro-Gly-Pro-Phe (using the abbreviated forms). Surprisingly, then, this plant source peptide compares very closely to the animal-derived beta-casomorphin BCM-7: Tyr - Pro - Phe - Pro - Gly - Pro - Ile. Notably, both peptides begin with a tyrosine followed by a proline, have a glycine or phenylalanine in the third location, and both have a total of 3 prolines each. Both gliadorphin and BCM-7 are therefore strong opiates, and are very stable. And, as Woodford points out, these two morphin peptides 'hunt together'.

The four scientists that stand out in this special field of inquiry are Robert Cade, Zhongjie Sun, Paul Shattock, and Kalle Reichelt. Cade and Sun were researchers at the University of Florida, Shattock was from the Autism Research Unit at the University of Sunderland, and Reichelt was from the Pediatrics Research Institute at the University of Oslo. Dr. Cade, who is

62

famous as the inventor of 'Gatorade', died on November 16th, 2007 ... much of his work has been carried on by his colleague, Dr. Sun.

These three groups have interacted together, and a number of their studies have been published in the journals *Nutritional Neuroscience*, *Autism*, and *Brain Dysfunction*. The key concept underlining their work is that many of the symptoms of neurological dysfunction are related to what we eat and how we metabolize what we eat. Particular foods that they have targeted include the two proteins, gluten and casein, and the opioid peptides that these two proteins are able to generate. They have shown that residues of gliadorphin and BCM-7 consistently show up in the urine of autistic children. They also report remarkable success with diets that are free of gluten and casein.

One intriguing piece of support to the BCM-7 association with neurological disorders was presented by none other than the New Zealand Dairy Board. By way of some in-depth investigation and probing, Keith Woodford was able to retrieve their application for a patent to supply A2 milk, presented in 2001. The application was entitled *Milk containing beta-casein with proline at position 67 does not aggravate neurological disorders*. The wording of this application is critical to the over-all credibility of the entire A1/A2 hypothesis, and sheds light on the mischievous switch by Fonterra later on to disavow the same hypothesis. Keep in mind that the Dairy Board, in essence, became Fonterra, and the same people were the key players then and afterwards. For example, Jeremy Hill was a co-author of several studies while with the Dairy Board, including at least two with Robert Elliot, and later became the 'Chief of Technology' for Fontera. I have included the abstract in whole:

'The invention is based on the discovery that the consumption of milk which contains a beta-casein-variant which has histidine or any other amino acid not proline at position 67, may on digestion cause the release

63

of an opioid which may induce or aggravate a neurological/mental disorder such as autism or Asperger's syndrome. The invention is supplying milk or milk products that contain beta-casein with proline at position 67 to susceptible individuals." (*Devil In The Milk,* pp 135)

How do opioid beta-casomorphins promote disease conditions ??

So ... how *do* opiates contribute to disease conditions ?? Wang et al, in their 2008 paper entitled *Opiate abuse, innate immunity, and bacterial infectious diseases,* explains that opiates can damage immune defenses that are essential for carrying out rapid immune reactions to invading pathogens. They state that:

"In vitro studies with innate immune cells from experimental animals and humans and in vivo studies with animal models have shown that opiate abuse impairs innate immunity and is responsible for increased susceptibility to bacterial infection." (Wang et al, 2008).

A number of other recent studies have suggested associations with opiate consumption and a variety of disease conditions. Noel et al (2008) reviewed the effects of opiates on the immune system and its effect on HIV replication and the progress of AIDS. Howard et al (2010) found evidence to indicate that opiate use among women with or at risk for HIV is associated with increased risk for diabetes.

Research has also implicated the BCM-7 molecule in impaired learning of infants and young children. Dubynin et al (2008) tested the effect of several opioid peptides on the learning ability of albino rat pups, and found that the BCM-7 peptide had a significant negative effect.

A recent Russian study by Kost et al (Kost, 2009) found that babies fed with cow's milk based formula containing BCM-7 demonstrated significant delay in psychomotor development. Another study in 2009 by Zozulia and his research group found that a dose of the BCM-7 peptide altered standard behavior response tests (the head-twitch test) in mice, which effect was blocked by subsequent application of the opioid suppressant drug, naloxone. Their conclusion was: "Thus, the influence of casomorphins on the serotoninergic system in vivo has been demonstrated for the first time." (Zozulia, 2009)

Although these studies add substantial credibility to the hypothesis that the BCM-7 peptide is associated with neurological function, there is a great need for additional high quality studies to be undertaken.

Milk allergy, milk intolerance, celiac disease, Crohn's disease, ulcerative colitis, sudden-death-syndrome, multiple sclerosis, and Parkinson's disease

Keith Woodford, in *Devil In The Milk*, explores the possible connection of BCM-7 and other beta-casomorphins with a number of additional disease conditions. He examines each in detail, and his statements and conclusions are compelling. However, what we now know about the possible link of beta-casomorphins, particularly BCM-7, with disease conditions such as milk allergy, milk intolerance, celiac disease, Crohn's disease, ulcerative colitis, sudden-death-syndrome, multiple sclerosis, and Parkinson's disease is sketchy, and highly conjectural. Some of these conditions relate to the condition of a 'leaky gut', and are therefore associated more with the process of how beta-casomorphins can enter the body that with their effect once in the body. Some conditions suggest that an auto-immune response is involved. Others that an oxidative process is at play. Or that an unknown neurological dysfunction in the brain is related, possibly caused by the strong opiate property of the beta-casomorphins.

Keith Woodford proposes that we take the BCM-7 hypothesis seriously, and to consider the 'big picture':

> "What we do know for sure is that for each disease there is one or more environmental trigger. We also know that milk keeps coming up as a prime candidate. If milk contains the cause then it almost certainly has to be one or more bioactive proteins in the milk. It is also likely that opioids are involved. It is hard to go past BCM-7 as a likely candidate. ... Undoubtedly there will be false leads, and the answers will be complex. It seems to me that BCM-7 is leaving enough tell-tale signs that it is eventually going to be unmasked as a villain. Surely it would be better that our milk was free of this devil." (pp 158)

Current Milk Production and the BCM-7 Peptide

In summary, the dairy cow carries the gene that determines its casein variant on the sixth chromosome. These variants can be divided into the A1, B, C, F, G, and H variants which have a histidine at position 67 and can therefore produce the BCM-7 peptide ... and the A2, A3, D, and E variants which have a proline at position 67 and therefore cannot produce the BCM-7 peptide. The proline at position 67 is the original variant ... the histidine at that position is theoretically due to a mutation that occurred with a specific breed in Europe several thousand years ago.

Dairy breeds vary greatly in respect to their casein variant, but for the 6 most common breeds in Western countries, the Holstein-Freisian is the most likely to produce milk with the BCM-7 molecule. The next most likely are the Ayrshire, Jersey, and Milking Shorthorn, which can all be ranked as equal. The next least likely is the Brown Swiss, and then the Guernsey is the least likely of all. There are also a number of breeds that are more specific to one locality, and these breeds are often of the A2, D, and E variant. Two interesting examples are the 'Normande' breed of France and the 'Icelandic Cow' or 'Norske' of Iceland. Both the French and Icelandic breeds are historically ancient, with little or no prior inter-breeding with dairy cattle from other countries. India is another example of a country that has a number of exotic dairy breeds; many of which also belong to the A2, D, and E variant group. It is noteworthy that Finland consumes the highest per capita amount of cow's milk, which is almost all Type A1 or contaminated with A1, and has the highest incidences of childhood diabetes.

For the sake of convenience, and because the majority of the A1, B, C, F, G, and H casein variants being produced worldwide today is A1 and B, we can simply call this group 'A1/B', or even just 'A1'. Similarly, we can shorten the A2, A3, D, and E group to 'A2'.

The prevalence of breeds in the dairy stock of individual counties varies greatly, as does the total cow population. In this respect New Zealand stands out. With a total human population of 4.23 million in 2007, the total dairy cow population was almost the same ... a whopping 4.20 million ... one dairy cow for every member of the population. The national dairy herd in 2007 was made up of 47% Holstein-Friesian, 15% Jersey, 2% Ayrshire, and the rest a mixture of Guernsey, Brown Swiss, and Meuse Rhine Issel.

The Holstein-Friesian is a magnificent milking animal. They are large, stylish animals with color patterns of black and white, or sometimes red and white. A mature cow weighs about 1,500 pounds and stands about 58 inches tall at the shoulder. Average annual production per animal in 2009 was 23,151 pounds of milk, 842 pounds of butterfat, and 711 pounds of protein. Top producing Holstein-Friesians are milked three times a day and have been known to produce in excess of 72,000 pounds of milk in 365 days. In the United States, more than 19 million

67

Holstein-Friesians are registered in the American Holstein Association's Herdbook, and account for more than 90% of the total dairy stock in the U.S.

As mentioned, the dairy cow carries the gene that determines its casein variant on the sixth chromosome. If we simplify the variants to A1 or A2, the trait for whether a cow will produce A1 or A2 beta casein is carried in the genes it inherits from its mother and father ... one gene is inherited from each parent for the trait of beta casein production, and thus each cow carries two genes determining what form of beta casein it produces. Cows can have only the A1 or only the A2 production trait, or they can have one of each.

As explained, the breed of the cow also plays an important role in this respect. For example, in the Holstein-Friesian, the most common trait distribution is:

• A quarter of the cows will carry traits for the production of A1 beta-casein, without the trait for A2, and will therefore produce only A1 milk.

• Half of the cows will carry a combination of traits for the production of both A1 and A2 beta-casein, and their milk will therefore be a 50 – 50 mix of A1 and A2.

• A quarter of the cows will carry traits for the production of A2 beta-casein, without the trait for A1, and will therefore produce only A2 milk.

This means, then, that 25% of milk from the Holstein-Friesian will be A1, 50% a 50 -50 mix of A1 and A2, and 25% only A2. However, unless care is taken to separate the pure A2 from the A1 and mixed A1/A2 milk, which is not normally done, the milks will be mixed in the holding tanks both at the farm and at the dairy. This then means that just about 100% of the mixed milk produced by the Holstein-Friesian will contain at least some A1 beta casein and will have the potential to produce the BCM-7 peptide. The exception will possibly be milk that is specifically kept separate from the bulk of the milk coming from the farms. However, there is no effort in the U.S. or Europe at the present time to identify and/or to separate the two variants of milk. This is only being done in New Zealand and Australia, and even in those countries only on a small scale. Much of this effort has been initiated by A2 Corporation, which has patents and copyrights involving A2 milk testing and distribution. One issue that has emerged is the difficulty in accurately testing milk and the dairy cow for A2 purity, and, secondly, guaranteeing that any milk that is sold in the marketplace as A2 is genuinely free of A1 contamination.

Woodford reports that in 2007 A2 milk was made available in 'Hy-Vee' supermarkets in seven mid-western states in the U.S. But in December, 2008 the A2 Milk Company announced that they were withdrawing A2 products from sale pending a new marketing strategy. There is currently no A2 milk commercially available in the United States. The A2 milk was "certified to contain at least 2 grams of A2 type beta-casein per serving". This implies that *not all the beta-casein was variant A2*, and so our BCM-7 devil could still be lurking in that glass of so-called A2 milk purchased at the Hy-Vee supermarket.

With 90% of the dairy cattle in the US being Holstein-Friesian, combined with the universal practice of mixing milks in holding tanks, almost all the milk currently sold commercially in the United States contains some A1, with the likelihood of it containing at least 50% A1.

An agreement between A2 Corporation and Purmil of Korea to market A2 milk in that country under the label 'Lotte' was terminated in December, 2009.

69

Summary of the Type A1/A2 Milk and BCM-7 Hypothesis

The case for the A1/A2 milk (BCM-7) hypothesis begins and ends with the scientific evidence, with perhaps an additional touch of logical inference. In summary, the evidence supporting the hypothesis can be divided into 10 different arguments:

1. The epidemiological evidence that demonstrates a remarkably high correlation between consumption of A1 versus A2 milk and the incidence of both Type 1 diabetes (IDDM) and ischaemic heart disease (IHD). The studies by Elliott and McLachlan stand out is this respect. The more specific comparisons of the populations of Finland versus France and Iceland, the Samoan children living in New Zealand versus their home country, and the Masai and Samburu people of Kenya, each add compelling examples.

2. The fact that BCM-7 is generated only from A1 beta-casein. A1 and A2 beta-casein are digested differently because of the histidine at position 67 instead of a proline, and therefore generate very different peptides, with very different properties.

3. The fact that BCM-7 caso-morphin can enter the body (a) under permeable stomach and small intestine lining conditions (ie. infants), (b) or under 'leaky gut' conditions, (c) plus evidence that it can enter even under normal conditions either after truncation by the enzyme 'dipeptidyl peptidase 4' (DPP4), located on the intestine lining, or at the position known as Caco-2 on the intestinal lining.

4. The fact that the BCM-7 peptide is an opioid beta-casomorphin, is a strong oxidant, and the amino acid composition is identical in the final four positions to the GLUT 2 molecule in the pancreas beta-cell. Each of these properties help explain the promotion of specific disease conditions.

5. The finding that mice and rats fed A1 beta-casein have a higher incidence of Type 1 diabetes (IDDM).

6. Evidence that rabbits fed on alternate diets of A1 versus A2 milk developed greater accumulations of arterial plaque (atherosclerosis) within the aorta artery.

7. The evidence that autistic and schizophrenic children typically excrete a large amount of BCM-7 in their urine, whereas normal children do not.

8. Identification of specific mechanisms whereby BCM-7 can (a) promote an auto-immune attack on pancreas beta-cells, (b) act as a strong oxidant on LDL, and (c) can pass through the blood-brain barrier and act as an opioid to promote neurological dysfunction.

9. The finding that persons with certain disease conditions often and consistently contain antibodies for BCM-7 in their bloodstream.

10. The extensive anecdotal evidence (testimonials) from persons who have switched to A2 milk and report improvements in a number of disease conditions.

References For Chapter Two

Aschaffenburg, R.; *Inherited casein variants in cow's milk*, Nature, 1961, November 4; 192:431-2

Aschaffenburg, R. *Inherited casein variants in cow's milk. II. Breed differences in the occurrence of β-casein variants*, Dairy Research, 1963, 30:251

Aschaffenburg, R.; *Variants of milk proteins and their pattern of inheritance*, J. of Dairy Science, 1965, January, 48:128- 32

Beales, P.E.; Elliott, R.B.; Flohe', S.; Hill, J.P.; Kolb, H.; Pozzilli,P.; Wang, G.S.; Wasmuth, H.; Scott, F.W.; *A multi-centre, blinded international trial of the effect of A1 and A2 β-casein variants on diabetes incidence in two rodent models of spontaneous Type 1 diabetes,* Diabetologia, 2002, Vol. 45, No. 9, September

Birgisdottir, B.E.; Hill, J.P.; Thorsson, A.V.; Thorsdottir, I.; *Lower consumption of cow milk protein A1 beta-casein at 2 years of age, rather than consumption among 11- to 14-year old adolescents, may explain the lower incidence of type 1 diabetes in Iceland than in Scandinavia,* Annals of Nutrition and Metabolism, 2008; 50(3): 177-83

Birgisdottir, B.E.; Hill, J.P.; Thorsdottir, I.; *Variations in consumption of cow milk proteins and lower incidence of Type 1 diabetes in Iceland vs the other 4 Nordic countries,* Diabetes, Nutrition & Metabolism - Clinical & Experimental, 2002, August; 15(4): 240-5

Cade, R.; Privette, M.; Fregly, M.; Rowland, N.; Sun, Z.; Zele, V.; Wagemaker, H.; Edelstein, C.; *Autism and schizophrenia: intestinal disorders,* Nutritional Neuroscience, 2000; 3:57-72

Cavallo, M.G.; Fava, D.; Monetini, L.; Pozzilli, P.; *Cell-mediated immune response to beta casein in recent-onset insulin-dependent diabetes: implications for disease pathogenesis,* Lancet, 1996, October 5; 348(9032): 926-8. This was a clinical study of 47 patients with recent-onset IDDM and 36 healthy controls. Interpretation: "The association between IDDM and early consumption of cow's milk may be explained by the generation of a specific immune response to beta casein. Exposure to cows' milk triggers a cellular and humoral anti-beta casein immune response which may cross-react with a beta-cell antigen. It is of interest that sequence homologies exist between beta casein and several beta-cell molecules."

Dr. Paolo Pozzilli is Professor of Diabetes and Clinical Research at the Centre for Diabetes at Barts and The London School of Medicine & Dentistry, London , and Professor of Endocrinology & Metabolic Diseases at the University Campus Bio-Medico in Rome , Italy.

He is the Delegate for University Campus Bio-Medico, Permanent Conference of Rectors of the Italian Universities (CRUI), Member Scientific Advisory Board, Graduate School in Molecular Medicine, University of Ulm and Member

Advisory Board, International Diabetes Federation, Group for Diabetes in the Youth. He coordinates the International PhD programme in Endocrinology and Metabolic Diseases between Queen Mary University of London, University Campus Bio-Medico in Rome and the University of Ulm, Germany.

Dr. Pozzilli is also the European Editor of Diabetes Metabolism Research & Reviews and Associate Editor of Nutrition Metabolism and Cardiovascular Disease. He is the Review Editor for the International Diabetes Monitor and Member of the International Commission of the Italian Society of Endocrinology.

He was the recipient of several awards amongst which the Andrew Cudworth Memorial Prize of the British Diabetic Association (1986), the G.B. Morgagni Prize, Young Investigator Award of the European Association of Metabolism (1989), the SID Prize 1994 (Italian Society of Diabetes), the Karol Marcinkowski Medal of the "Poznan Academy of Medicine"(1997), the Mary Jane Kugel Award, Juvenile Diabetes Research Foundation, USA (2003 and 2006) and the Diabetes Honoris Causa, Paulescu Foundation & Romanian Society of Diabetes (2007).

Dr Pozzilli is involved with a wide assortment of studies in the field of diabetes, including animal studies and the use of stem cell therapy.

Chin, D.; Ng-Kwai-Hang, K.F.; *Application of mass spectrometry for the identification of genetic variants of milk proteins,* in "Milk Protein Polymorphism", International Dairy Federation, Brussels, Belgium, Special Issue no. 9702: 334- 339, 1997

Chung, E.R.; Han, S.K.; Rhim, T.J.; *Milk protein polymorphisms as genetic marker in Korean native cattle,* Asian-Australasian Journal of Animal Sciences, 1995; 8:187-194

De Noni, I.; *Release of β-casomorphins 5 and 7 during simulated gastro-intestinal digestion of bovine β-casein variants and milk-based infant formula.* Food Chemistry, 2008, October 15; Vol. 110, Issue 4: 897-903

Dohan, C.F.; *Cereals and schizophrenia: data and hypothesis,* Acta Psychiatrica Scandinavica, 1966; 42:125-152

Dohan, C.F. et al; *Relapsed schizophrenics: more rapid improvement on a milk and cereal free diet.* British Journal of Psychiatry, 1969; 115:595-596

Dohan, C.F.; *Is celiac disease a clue to pathogenesis of schizophrenia?* Journal of Mental Hygiene, 1969; 53:525-529

Dohan, C.F. et al; *Is schizophrenia rare if grain is rare?* Journal of Biology and Psychiatry, 1984; 19(3):385-399

Dong, C.; Ng-Kwai-Hang, K.F.; *Characterization of a non-electrophoretic genetic variant of β-casein by peptide mapping and mass spectrometric analysis,* International Dairy Journal; 8:967-972

Dubynin, V.A.; Malinovskala, I.V.; Beliaeva, IuA.; Stovolosov, I.S.; Bespalova, ZhD.; Andreeva, L.A.; Kamenskil, A.A.; Miasoedov, N.F.; *Delayed effect of exorphins on learning of albino rat pups,* Izv Akad Nauk Ser Biol, 2008, Jan-Feb; (1): 53-60

Elliott, R.B.; *Diabetes – A man made disease,* Medical Hypotheses, 2006, Vol. 67, Issue 2: 388-91

Elliott, R.B.; Harris, D.P.; Hill, J.P.; Bibby, N.J.; Wasmuth, H.E.; *Type 1 (insulin-dependent) diabetes mellitus and cow milk: casein variant consumption,* Diabetologia, 1999, March; 42(3): 292-6. This was the preliminary study to the Laugesen and Elliott study of 2003.

Elliott, R.B.; Laugesen, M.; *The influence of consumption of A1 β-casein on heart disease and Type 1 diabetes – the authors reply*, The New Zealand Medical Journal, 2003, March; Vol. 116, No. 1179

Elliott, R.B.; Martin, J.M.; *Dietary protein: a trigger of insulin-dependent diabetes in the BB rat?* Diabetologia, 1984; 26: 297-99.

Fava, D.; Leslie, R.D.; Pozzilli, P.; *Relationship between dairy product consumption and incidence of IDDM in childhood in Italy,* Diabetes Care, 1994, December; 17(12): 1488-90. This is an early study by Pozzilli and his group on the relationship

74

between dairy product consumption and the incidence of IDDM, before they had investigated the BCM-7 peptide.

Formaggioni, A.; Summer, A.; Malacarne, M.; Mariani, P.; *Milk Protein Polymorphism: Detection and Diffusion of the Genetic Variants in Bos Genus,* Instituto di Zootecnica, Alimentazione e Nutrizione, Universita degli Studi, 1999. www.unipr.it/arpa/facvet/annali/1999/formaggioni/formaggioni.

Gepts, W.; *Pathologic anatomy of the pancreas in juvenile diabetes mellitus,* British Medical Journal, 1965, November 03, 4(5887):260-262

Glarum, M.; Robinson, B.H.; Martini, J.M.; *Could bovine serum albumin be the initiating antigen ultimately responsible for the development of insulin-dependent diabetes mellitus?* Diabetes Research, 1989, March; 10(3): 103-7. Conclusion: "Analysis of the amino-acid homology in relation to the DR/DQ allotypes found in the human population gave a strong correlation between the combined DR and DQ homology score with bovine serum albumin and the incidence of IDDM."

Han, S.K.; Chung, E.Y.; Lee, K.M.; *Studies on the genetic polymorphism of milk proteins in Korean Cattle,* Proceeding of the 5th World Conference of Animal Production, Tokyo, Japan, August 14-19, 1983; 2:51-52

Han, S.K.; Shin, Y.C.; *Biochemical characterization of the new β-casein variant in Korean Cattle,* Proceedings XXVth International Conference on Animal Genetics, Tours, France, 1996, July 21-24; 144

Henschen, A.; Lottspeich, F.; Branti, V.; Teschemacher, H.; *Novel opioid peptides derived from casein (beta-casomorphins), II. Structure of active components from bovine casein peptone,* Hoppe-Seyler's Zeitschrift fur physiologische Chemie, 1979, September; 360(9): 1217-24.

Howard, A.A.; Hoover, D.R.; Anastos, K.; Wu, X.; Shi, Q.; Strickler, H.D.; Cole, S.R.; Cohen, M.H.; Kovacs, A.; Augenbraun, M.; Latham, P.S.; Tien, P.C.; *The effects of opiate use and hepatitis C virus infection on risk of diabetes mellitus in the women's interagency HIV study.,* Journal of

Acquired Immune Deficiency Syndromes, 2010, June; 54(2): 152-9

Iwan, M.; Jarmolowska, B.; Bielikowicz, K.; Kostyra, E.; Kostyra, H.; Kaczmarski, M.; *Transport of micro-opioid receptor agonists and antagonis peptides across Caco-2 monolayer,* Peptides, 2008, June; 29(6); 1042-7.

Kaminski, S.; Cieslinska, A.; Kostyra, E.; *Polymorphism of bovine beta-casein and its potential effect on human health,* Journal of Applied Genetics, 2007; 48(3):189-98. This review also acknowledges the Type A1/A2 milk and BCM-7 hypothesis and suggests that further in-depth research is needed.

Karges, W.; Hammond-McKibben, D.; Gaedigk, R.; Shibuya, N.; Cheung, R.; Dosch, H.M.; *Loss of self-tolerance to ICA69 in non-obese diabetic mice,* Diabetes, 1997, October; 46(10): 1548-56. This study confirms that T-cell response to both pancreatic beta-cell antigens and milk proteins can demonstrate mimicry. This supports the hypothesis that an auto immune response may inadvertently attack both a milk protein peptide and the pancreatic beta-cells.

Karjaleinen, J.; Martin, J.M.; Knip, M.; Ilonen, J.; Robinson, B.H.; Savilahtl, E.; Akerblom, H.K.; Dosch, H.M.; *A bovine albumin peptide as a possible trigger of insulin-dependent diabetes mellitus.* New England Journal of Medicine, 1992, July 30; 327(5): 302-7

Kiddy, C.A.; Peterson, R.F.; Kopfler, F.C.; *Genetic control of the variants of β-casein A,* J. of Dairy Science, 49, 742, 1966

Klemetti, P.; *T-Cell Mediated Immunity in the Pathogenesis of Insulin-Dependent Diabetes Mellitus,* PhD. Dissertation for the University of Helsinki, November, 1999

Knip, M.; Virtanen, S.M.; Seppa, K.; Lionen, J.; Savilahti, E.; Vaarala, O.; Reunanen, A.; Teramo, K.; Hamalainen, A.; Paronen, J.; Dosch, H.; Hakulinen, T.; Akerblom, H.; *Dietary Intervention in Infancy and Later Signs of Beta-Cell Autoimmunity*, for the Finnish TARIGR Study Group, New England Journal of Medicine, 2010, Nov 11, 363: 1900- 1908

Kost, N.V.; Sokolov, O.Y. Kurasova, O.B.; Dimitriev, A.D.; Tarakanova, J.N.; Gabaeva, M.V.; Zolotarev, Y.A.; Dadayan, A.K.; Grachev, S.A.; Korneeva, E.V.; Mikheeva, I.F.; Zozulya, A.A.; *Beta-casomorphins-7 in infants on different type of feeding and different levels of psychomotor development.* Peptides, 2009, October; 30(10): 1854-60

Laugesen, M.; Elliot, R.; *Ischaemic heart disease, Type 1 diabetes, and cow milk A1 beta-casein,* New Zealand Medical Journal, 2003, January 24; 116(1168): U295. This is the study that finally drew attention to the A1, A2 milk variant and the BCM-7 molecule issue.

McLachlan, C.N.; *Beta-casein A1, ischaemic heart disease mortality, and other illnesses,* Medical Hypotheses, 2001, February; 56(2): 262-72

McLachlan, C.N.; Olson, F.; *Setting the record straight: A1 β-casein, heart disease and diabetes,* The New Zealand Medical Journal, 2003, March, Vol. 116, No. 1170

Meisel, H.; FitzGerald, R.J.; *Opioid peptides encrypted in intact milk protein sequences,* British Journal of Nutrition, 2000; 84, Suppl. 1, S27-S31.

Ng-Kwai-Hang, K.F.; Hayes, J.F.; Moxley, J.E.; Monardes, H.G.; *Association of genetic variants of casein and milk serum proteins with milk, fat, and protein production by dairy cattle,* Journal of Dairy Science, 1984, April; 67(4): 835-40.

Ng-Kwai-Hang, K.F.; Grosclaude, F.; *Genetic polymorphism of milk proteins,* Chapter 16 of *Advance Dairy Chemistry*, pp 737-814, Fox, P.F. and McSweeney, P.L.H.; editors; published by Kluwer Academic/Plenum Publishers, New York, 2002

Noel, R.J. Jr; Rivera-Amill, V.; Buch, S.; Kumar, A.; *Opiates, immune system, acquired immunodeficiency syndrome, and nonhuman primate model,* Journal of Neurovirol, 2008, August; 14(4): 279-85.

Peterson, R.F; Kopfler, F.C.; *Detection of new types of β-casein by polyacrylamide gel electrophoresis at acid pH: a proposed nomenclature,* Biochemical and Biophysical Research Communications, 22, 388-392, 1966

Reichelt, K. et al; *Biologically active peptide-containing fractions in schizophrenia and childhood autism,* Advances in Biochemical Psychopharmacology, 1981; 28:627-647

Reichelt, K. et al; *Gluten, milk proteins and autism: dietary intervention effects on behavior and peptide secretions,* Journal of Applied Nutrition, 1990; 42:1-11

Scott, F.; Kolb, H.; *A1 β-casein milk and Type 1 diabetes: causal relationship probed in animal models,* New Zealand Medical Journal, 2003, March; Vol. 116, No. 1170

Shattock, P.; Kennedy, A.; Rowell, F.; Berney, T.; *Role of neuropeptides in autism and their relationships with classical transmitters,* Brain Dysfunction, 1990, 3:328-46

Sidor, K.; Jarmolowska, B.; Kaczmarski, M.; Kostyra, E.; Iwan, M.; Kostyra, H.; *Content of beta-casomorphins in milk of women with a history of allergy,* Pediatric Allergy and Immunology, 2008, November; 19(7): 587-91.

Sienkiewicz-Szlapka, S.; Jarmolowska, B.; Krawczuk, H.; Bielkowicz, K.; *Transport of bovine milk-derived opioid peptides across a Caco-2 monolayer,* International Dairy Journal, 2009, April; Vol. 19, Issue 4: 252-57

Steinerova, A.; Stozik, F.; Racek, J.; Tatzbar, F.; Zima, T.; Stetina, R.; *Antibodies against Oxidized LDL in infants.* Clinical Chemistry, 2001; 47: 1137-8

Sun, Z.; Cade, J.R.; Fregly, M.J.; Privette, R.M.; *Beta-casomorphin induces Fos-like immunoreactivity in discrete brain regions relevant to schizophrenia and autism,* Autism, 1999, 3(1): 67-81

Taliford, K.A.; Berry, C.L.; Thomas, A.C.; Campbell, J.H.; *A casin variant in cow's milk is atherogenic,* Atherosclerosis, 2003, September; 170(1): 11-2. Sixty rabbits were divided into 10 groups and fed different concentrations of A1 and A2 beta-caseins. The rabbits fed the A1 variant beta-casein had significantly higher concentrations of arterial plaque.

Conclusion: "It is concluded that beta-casein A1 is atherogenic compared with beta-casein A2."

Thompson, M.P.; Kiddy, C.A.; Johnston, J.O.; Weinberg, R.M.; *Genetic polymorphism in caseins of cow's milk. II. Confirmation of the genetic control of beta-casein variations,* Journal of Dairy Science; 47: 378-81, 1964.

Thorsdottir, I.; Birgisdottir, B.E.; Johannsdottir, I.M.; Harris, D.P.; Hill, J.; Steingrimsdottir, L.; Thorsson, A.V.; *Different β-caseub fractions in Icelandic versus Scandinavian cow's milk may influence diabetogenicity of cow's milk in infancy and explain low incidence of insulin-dependent diabetes mellitus in Iceland.* Pediatrics, 2000, 106(4): 719-24

Thorsdottir, I.; Reykdal, O.; *Food and the low incidence of IDDM in Iceland*, Scandivanvian Journal of Nutrition, Naringsforskning, 1997, 4: 97

Torreilles, J.; Guerin, M.C.; *Casein-derived peptides can promote human LDL oxidation by a peroxidase-dependent and metal-independent process.* Comptes Rendus des Seances de la Societe de Biologie et des ses Filiales (Paris), 1995; 189(5): 933-42

Van Eenenw, A.; Fernando-Medrano, J.; *Milk Protein Polymorphisms in California Dairy Cattle,* Journal of Dairy Sciences, Vol. 74, No. 5, 1991

Virtanen, S.M.; Rasanen, L.; Aro, A.; Lindstrom, J.; Sippola, H.; Lounamaa, R.; Toivanen, L.; Tuomilehto, J.; Akerblom, H.K.; *Infant feeding in Finnish children less than 7yr of age with newly diagnosed IDDM, Childhood Diabetes in Finland Study Group.* Diabetes Care, 1991, May, vol. 14, no. 5:415-417

Virtanen, S.M.; Rasanen, L.; Ylonen, K.; Aro, A.; Clayton, D.; Langholz, B.; Pitkaniemi, J.; Savilahti, E.; Lounamaa, R.; Tuomilehto, J.; Early introduction of dairy products associated with increased risk of IDDM in Finnish children. The Childhood Diabetes in Finland Study Group. Diabetes, 1993, December, vol. 42, no. 12:1786-1790

Virtanen, S.M.; Laara, E.; Hypponen, E.; Reijonen, H.; Rasanen, L.; Aro, A.; Knip, M.; Ilonen, J.; Akerblom, H.K.; *Cow's milk* consumption, *HLA-DQB1 genotype, and type a diabetes: a nested case-control study of siblings of children with diabetes. Childhood diabetes in Finland study group.* Diabetic Medicine, 1998, September, vol. 15, issue 9:730-738

Virtanen, S.M.; Hypponen, E.; Laara, E.; Vahasako, P.; Kulmala, P.; Savola, K.; Rasanen, L.; Aro, A.; Knip, M.; Akerblom, H.K.; *Cow's milk consumption, disease-associated autoantibodies and Type 1 diabetes mellitus: a follow-up study in siblings of diabetic children,* Diabetic Medicine, published online July 19, 2004

(Virtanen, S.M.); Knip, M.; Veijola, R.; Hyoty, H.; Vaarala, O.; Akerblom, H.K.; *Environmental Triggers and Determinants of Type 1 Diabetes,* Diabetes, 2005, December, vol. 54, no. suppl 2:S125-S136

Visser, S.; Slangen, C.J.; Rollema, H.S.; *Phenotyping of bovine milk proteins by reversed-phase high performance liquid chromatography,* Journal of Chromatography, 1991, 548:361-370

Visser, S.; Slangen, C.J.; Lagerwerf, F.M.; van Dongen, W.D.; Haverkamp, J.; *Identification of a new genetic variant of bovine β-casein using reversed-phase high-performance liquid chromatography and mass spectrometric analysis,* Journal of Chromatography A, 1995, 711:141-150

Wang, J.; Barke, R.A.; Ma, J.; Charboneau, R.; Roy, S.; *Opiate abuse, innate immunity, and bacterial infectious diseases,* Archivum Immunologiae Et Tharapiae Experimentalis, 2008, Sept-Oct; 56(5): 299-309.

Zozulia, A.A.; Meshavkin, V.K.; Sokolov Olu; Kost, N.V.; *(Naloxone-induced suppression of the behavioral manifestation of serotoninergic system hperactivation by beta-casomorphin-7 in mice),* Eksp Klin Farmakol, 2009, Mar-Apri; 72(2): 3-5. A dose of the BCM-7 peptide to mice was shown to alter standard behavior response tests (the head-twitch test) in mice, which effect was blocked by subsequent application of the opioid suppressant drug, naloxone. Conclusion: "Thus, the influence of casomorphins on the serotoninergic system in vivo has been demonstrated for the first time."

Chapter Three

SO ... WHAT'S BEING DONE ABOUT IT ??

The Problem Becomes Two

It may not be so much a question of what science will eventually conclude ... although this is extremely important ... but may be more a matter of consumers knowing the truth, being protected, and having a choice.

What is at stake is not only a challenge to the dairy industry, but, much more importantly, is your and my health ... and the health of our babies and our children ... and of generations to come. And what about the increasing millions who suffer and will suffer from diabetes, heart disease, and neurological disorders.

The New Zealand Dairy Board and the New Zealand Dairy Research Institute

That fateful day in 1993 when Jeremy Hill explained the genetic-based difference between Types A1 and A2 cow's milk to Robert Elliot, a key piece to the BCM-7 puzzle was put in place, and became a catalyst for continued research by Elliot and a number of other scientists. Jeremy Hill was a research scientist with the New Zealand Dairy Research Institute (NZDRI) at the time. The NZDRI was the research arm of the New Zealand Dairy Board (NZDB), which was a giant government co-op for almost the entire New Zealand dairy industry. It is important to note that Jeremy Hill was a co-researcher in many of the studies that followed, notably with Elliot, Thorsdottir, and Birgisdottir More about this below.

The basic stance that the New Zealand Dairy Board decided to take on the Type A1 beta-casein issue was evident as far back as 1997. Even back then there was enough information and concern circulating among board members to warrant a group-wide decision. They needed to decide on whether or not to initiate breeding techniques to switch New Zealand's dairy herds from mainly Type A1 milk producers to Type A2 producers. It is important to note that the New Zealand dairy industry took the research on the Type A1/A2 and BCM-7 hypothesis very seriously, even at that early stage of research development, and took it seriously enough to initiate a country-wide program to convert the dairy herds away from Type A1 production to Type A2-only production. Keith Woodford explains that he was able to obtain unpublished documents from the New Zealand Dairy Group and the New Zealand Dairy Research Institute related to the industry's discussions at that time. He reports this information in his paper to the International Diabetes Federation (IDF) Congress, in 2008. The documents reveal that it was a close decision for the NZDB members. The challenge at hand would be first to convert the herds, which could be a ten-year-long process or even more, and secondly the problem of how to protect the market for the continuing A1 milk being produced, and also to create a market for the new type A2 milk. The challenge, and the cost, would be formidable. The decision by the NZ Dairy Board at the time was to do nothing overt, especially not to cause concern among the public, and to work behind-the-scenes in anticipation of a future shift in demand away from Type A1 milk in favor of Type A2. (Woodford, 2008)

Fonterra

New Zealand is truly a 'land of milk and honey'! Annual production of honey exceeds 11,000 tons ... with a population of only 4.2 million, that equals about 5.8 pounds per capita per year. And how about milk? ... Well, New Zealand is the home of one dairy cow for each man, woman, and child in the country, and produces over 15 million tons of milk per year ... or about 3.6 tons per person. Dairy is New Zealand's largest industry and its biggest export earner.

The dairy industry in New Zealand has traditionally been characterized by a large number of individual dairy farms, usually small family-owned operations, which join collectively in co-ops to market their products. Prior to 2001 the N.Z. farmers were united under the New Zealand Dairy Board, with all but a very few of the dairy farms in the nation joined in one marketing cooperative. But the decision to deregulate in that year resulted in the formation of Fonterra Cooperative Group Ltd., with 10,500 individual farms, or 95% of the total N.Z. farms. Westland Co-operative Dairy Company and Tatua Cooperative Dairy Company Ltd. elected not to join Fonterra, and made up the remaining 5%.

Fonterra has been a success story, expanding rapidly since 2001, and has now become a major player in the global dairy industry. The latest statistics rank Fonterra as the fifth largest dairy company in the world ... and the largest milk processor. Ninety-five percent of New Zealand's milk and milk product production is exported. This amount significantly affects the total global picture. While New Zealand's milk production accounts for only 2% of world production, it accounts for 33% of world trade in dairy products. Key products include cheeses, protein concentrates, and biomedical and biohealth products. It is estimated that Fonterra currently controls, directly or indirectly, as much as 40% of the world's dairy industry.

Fonterra and Type A1, A2 milk

Before deregulation in 2001, and for some time afterwards, the N.Z. mainstream dairy industry was keenly interested in the A1/A2 hypothesis, as mentioned. This was largely due to the studies by Robert Elliot and Jeremy Hill, and the influence of Corran McLachlan. For example, the New Zealand Dairy Board was a co-applicant on a patent in the year 2000 which cited an association of type A1 milk with diabetes, and another one in 2001 which cited an association with autism. Jeremy Hill authored several reports to support these patent applications. A copy of one of the reports was given to Howard Paterson (A2 Corporation). In this report Jeremy Hill acknowledged the science and data in support of the Type A1/A2 hypothesis, and included some research of his own. When Fonterra was formed in 2001 Dr. Hill became Group Director of Technology for Fonterra's equivalence to the NZDRI, called the Fonterra Research Centre. In 2006 Jeremy Hill was also co-author of at least three Icelandic studies which linked A1 milk consumption and Type 1 diabetes.

Prior to deregulation the New Zealand Dairy Board, which also administered the national dairy cattle breeding system, had decided to test the A1/A2 status of all the dairy bulls. A strong interest in the conversion had continued to emerge. Woodford reports that as of 2005 approximately 500 N.Z. farmers were in the process of converting to A2 production.

Before the year 2005 Fonterra sought patents similar to, and in competition with those being applied for by A2 Corporation. On July 4th, 2005, the Intellectual Property Office of New Zealand made a momentous decision on which entity was to obtain the patent rights, and ruled against Fonterra and in favor of A2 Corporation on all matters pertaining to the patent applications by both companies.

84

The 'Great Debate'

A2 Corporation had been at odds with the New Zealand Dairy Board from the beginning of its conception. It is not clear just when the NZDB first decided to stand up against A2 Corporation, but Woodford suggests that it was probably soon after the fateful meeting in October, 2000, between Howard Paterson of A2 Corporation and Warren Larson, N.Z. Dairy Board Chief. Woodford reports:

> "It was at that meeting that phrases like 'class-action' started to be thrown about by Howard Paterson in relation to non-disclosure of key information. Warren Larsen was clearly concerned that A2 Corporation was a bunch of irresponsible cowboys that could put the New Zealand dairy industry at risk. They needed to be stopped in their tracks."

After the takeover by Fonterra, the animosity and competitiveness between Fonterra and A2 Corporation intensified. It was a curious situation. At that time Fonterra was supportive of the A1/A2 (BCM-7) hypothesis and was interested in obtaining the same sort of patents and copyrights as did A2 Corporation. The competitiveness over patents intensified, and outright animosity became the prevailing mood. The deaths of both Paterson and McLachlan in 2003 surely added to Fonterra's confidence that they would succeed over A2 Corporation in all aspects. The ruling by the Intellectual Property Office in favor of A2 Corporation in 2005 must have been a severe blow to Fonterra, and a turning point. From then on they were not only against A2 Corporation, but were against the entire A1/A2, BCM-7 hypothesis.

The ensuing debate is full of intrigue, mischief, and outright unethical science, plus the muscling of big business.

A key factor was clearly the untimely deaths of both Howard Paterson and Corran McLachland. Conspiracy advocates have jumped to the sensationalist conclusion that their deaths were

85

programmed by other interests, but Woodford reports otherwise. Howard Paterson was in Fiji on July 1, 2003 for a business meeting, but failed to show up. He was found dead in his hotel room, and the autopsy determined that he had, in fact, choked on some potato chips. He was 50 years old. Corran McLachlan had been fighting a losing battle with melanoma cancer for ten years, and died early in August 2003. He was 59.

The deaths of these two men could have meant the end of A2 Corporation, and the A1/A2 milk issue may have died with them. Indeed, the ensuing effort by Fonterra after taking the place of the New Zealand Dairy Board was aimed in that direction. The next segment of the unfolding story, again related by Woodford, is about Fonterra's counter attack and subsequent articles and studies that attempted to negate the A1/A2, BCM-7 hypothesis. It is again absorbing reading. Once more, I encourage the reader to read *Devil In The Milk.* For this part Dr. Woodford is not only a writer and a reporter, but is an investigating journalist and a scientist.

The FAD trial

Early in 2001 the New Zealand Dairy Board took the initiative to sponsor a large-scale international study to expand on Elliot's earlier work with rats and mice, to further test the association of A1 β-casein with diabetes. It is not clear whether the NZ Dairy Board was supportive of the A1/A2 milk (BCM-7) hypothesis in undertaking this study, or that they changed their position somewhere enroute. Never-the-less, the published results were highly negative.

The study was entitled *A multi-centre, blinded international trial of the effect of A1 and A2 β-casein variants on diabetes incidence in two rodent models of spontaneous Type 1 diabetes,* and was authored by nine scientists. Three of them are already known to this discussion: Robert Elliott, Jeremy Hill, and P. Pozzilli. The others were P.E Beales, R.B. Flohe', H. Kolb, G.S. Wang, H. Wasmuth, and F.W. Scott. Because Beales was the

86

first author named, the study has sometimes been called the Beales et al study. But Frazer Scott was the listed 'corresponding author' and is therefore assumed to be the team leader. As a whole the nine authors represented New Zealand, Canada, Great Britain, Germany, and Italy.

Three laboratories were set up: one in New Zealand, one in Canada, and one in Great Britain. Two rodent species were used: the BB mice, and the NOD rat, which are both known to be susceptible to diabetes. From the very beginning, the study had many flaws. The rodent species were not consistent, and the diets were complicated: four were based on a casein-based product called 'Pregestimil', four were based on a soy bean product called 'Prosobee', and one of the diets was a milk-free, cereal-based rodent diet. Both the Pregestimil and the Prosobee are human infant formulas produced and marketed by Mead Johnson. All the diets were prepared in New Zealand and distributed from there.

The study then encountered a series of problems. First, the New Zealand mice suffered from an outbreak of 'Clostridium disease' and many died. The New Zealand trial portion was therefore abandoned. This lab was under the supervision of Robert Elliott, who then stepped back as a primary player.

The second calamity was that the Pregetimil used was found to already have a high content of BCM-7. This fact was reported by Jeremy Hill in a document dated October, 2000. However, no mention of this was made in the final paper published in the journal Diabetologia in 2002, and it is not clear whether all the authors were aware of this fact. The importance of this is tantamount to invalidating the entire trial … it meant that a strong confounder was present, and that the data would also be invalid.

Woodford once again was the relentless pursuer, and he later contacted the various authors, scrutinized the data, and even went to battle with the journal, Diabetologia. Robert Elliot

87

reported that he was not aware of the Pregetimil contamination, and made the following statement in an email to Woodford:

"I am still upset by this news. Why did Jeremy do that?? If the Pregestimil used contained BCM-7 when the manufacturers state that no peptide (more than) 4 amino acids in length is present in their product, something odd has happened.

It of course invalidates the Pregestimil arm of the FAD study. This means that the two major conclusions of the FAD study are invalid." (*Devil In The Milk*, pp 106-7)

A great deal of cover-up, denials of responsibility, and a refusal to retract the study from Diabetologia ensued. Jeremy Hill denied that he had known about the Pregestimil contamination. Diabetologia even refused to investigate, or to print an acknowledgement that the study had been flawed. In a final heated communication with the editor, Woodford referred him to a much quoted editorial from the December, 2005 issue of New Scientist:

"Science runs on trust. Governments give researchers money on the understanding they will use it fairly and honestly report their results. Peer reviewers assume that what they are judging is a fair account of what happened; they are not yet charged with policing dubious data. Without trust the whole scientific world will collapse." (*Devil In The Milk*, pp 114)

It is interesting that Robert Elliot later joined with Keith Woodford in various communications and media presentations, and has consistently supported the A1/A2 milk (BCM-7) hypothesis, and has stated repeatedly that the FAD trial was flawed and the conclusions invalid. In addition, Woodford re-analyzed the FAD data, correcting for the contaminated Pregetimil, and concludes that the data do, in fact, support the correlation between the consumption of Type A1 beta-casein and an increased incidence of Type 1 diabetes.

Fraser Scott and Hubert Kolb, two of the FAD trial authors, later published a review entitled *A1 β-casein milk and Type 1 diabetes: causal relationship probed in animal models* in The New Zealand Medical Journal, March 2003. They repeated the same data and conclusions as the flawed FAD trial ... and of course they failed to mention that the Pregetimil feed was contaminated with BCM-7.

The 2004 Fonterra paper

It was clear that Fonterra was beginning to play both sides of the fence, even before the year 2003. But with the published studies by Elliott and Laugesen, and McLachlan, the A1/A2 BCM-7 hypothesis gained notice. The deaths of McLachlan and Paterson were certainly additional factors. But Fonterra's hopes to lead with the Type A1/A2 milk issue was dealt a deciding blow with the 2005 decision by the New Zealand Intellectual Property Office to rule in favor of A2 Corporation in all matters concerning related patents and property rights.

Early in 2004 Fonterra, even before the ruling of the Intellectual Property Office, began their counter-attack. A 12-page document was released (but never published) that set the groundwork for their assault. Woodford reports that this report "included many erroneous statements, and a number of quotes taken seriously out of context." (Woodford, 2008)

The New Zealand Food Safety Authority (NZFSA), and the Swinburn report

According to their website, the "New Zealand Food Safety Authority's mandate is to protect consumers by providing an effective food regulatory programme covering food produced and consumed in New Zealand as well as imports and exports of food products".

Its two-fold task, therefore, is the protection and promotion of public health and safety, and secondly the promotion and facilitation of access to markets for New Zealand food and food

89

products. In the past the agency worked closely with the New Zealand Ministry of Agriculture and Forestry (MAF) ... as of July, 2010 the New Zealand Food Safety Authority and MAF were joined as a single government regulation and monitoring agency.

Within days after the publication of Elliott and Laugesen's study in January, 2003, the NZFSA issued a press release entitled *Milk Still Part of Balanced Diet*. The release acknowledged Elliott and Laugesen's finding, but concluded:

> "The Ministry of Health supports the NZFSA's view that the evidence is not strong enough to change the health messages around milk or to require any special labeling on milk or milk products ... milk is nutritious and beneficial and should remain part of a balanced diet."
> (*Devil In The Milk*, pp 169)

By March, 2003, NZFSA was in negotiation with Dr. Boyd Swinburn from Deakin University in Australia to review the A1/A2 milk (BCM-7) hypothesis and to author a report. Swinburn was also the former Medical Director of the National Heart Foundation of New Zealand. Swinburn drafted his report within a couple of months, but the report was not released until August, 2004. There was a great deal of inside debate going on during this period, which Woodford reports and discusses in *Devil In The Milk*. Just before his death, Corran McLachlan was also involved, and Woodford reports that he was furious with NZFSA's decision to seek out a review study by Swinburn.

With publication of the report, NZFSA issued its own press release, stating:

> "There is no food safety issue with either type of milk ... Professor Swinburn's review shows that there is insufficient evidence to demonstrate benefits of one type of milk protein over another."

However, there was definitely some mischief at play. When NZFSA released Swinburn's report for publication, it was discovered that omissions and changes had been made to the report text. First, the 'Lay Summary' had been left out, which contained some conclusions that were contradictory to NZFSA's released statements. Plus, the length of the document had been shortened by omissions, and then 'stretched' by inserting extra spaces between paragraphs in an attempt to conceal the fact that omissions had been made. Interestingly, since the time of publication back in 2004, Keith Woodford has had numerous communications and meetings with Dr. Swinburn, and Dr. Swinburn has joined with Woodford in media presentations and written statements … he is actually very supportive of the A1/A2 milk (BCM-7) hypothesis, and is dismayed that the NZFSA has mis-represented his conclusions.

With heavy pressure from the media and Woodford, with Woodford being the prime motivator, the Lay Summary was finally released, and NZFSA even put it on its website … but the damage had been done, and the news was already old. Never-the-less, what the Lay Summary actually said is important, and so I am including the final three paragraphs (from *Devil In The Milk,* pp 174-5):

"The A1/A2 hypothesis is both intriguing and potentially very important for public health if it is proved correct. It should be taken seriously and further research is needed. In addition, the appropriate government agencies have a responsibility to communicate the current state of evidence to the public, including uncertainty about the evidence. Further public health actions, such as changing dietary advice or requiring labeling of milk products, are not considered to be warranted at this stage. Monitoring is also required to ensure that any claims made for A2 milk fall within the regulations for food claims.

Changing the dairy herds to more A2 producing cows is an option for the dairy and associated industries and these decisions will undoubtedly be made on a commercial basis. Changing dairy herds to more A2 producing cows may significantly improve public health, if the A1/A2 hypothesis is proved correct, and it is highly unlikely to do harm.

As a matter of individual choice, people may wish to reduce or remove A1 beta-casein from their diet (or their children's diet) as a precautionary measure. This may be particularly relevant for those individuals who have or are at risk of the diseases mentioned (Type 1 diabetes, coronary heart disease, autism and schizophrenia). However, they should do so knowing that there is substantial uncertainty about the benefits of such an approach."

Woodford tells us that Dr. Swinburn had argued with the NZFSA, including telling them in one communication that:

"… if I had a child with Type 1 diabetes and was due to have another and I could easily obtain and afford A2 milk or formula, I would certainly use it for the next child because the cost/benefit is low because of the potentially very large benefit of preventing Type 1 diabetes."

A copy of the Lay Summary to the report is now available online from the NZFSA website: www.nzfsa.govt.nz/policy-law/projects/a1-a2-milk/lay-summary.htm

A.S. Truswell; *The A2 milk case: a critical review*

This review was published in the European Journal of Clinical Nutrition, in November, 2005. It has been cited extensively by agencies and other scientists interested in discrediting the A1/A2 milk (BCM-7) hypothesis. It is worthwhile to present the entire abstract to the study, which is as follows:

"This review outlines a hypothesis that A1, one of the common variants of β-casein, a major protein in cow's milk, could facilitate the immunological processes that lead to type 1 diabetes (DM-1). It was subsequently suggested that A1 β-casein may also be a risk factor for coronary heart disease (CHD), based on between-country correlations of CHD mortality with estimated national consumption of A1 β-casein in a selected number of developed countries. A company, A2 Corporation, was set up in New Zealand in the late 1990s to test cows and market milk in several countries with only the A2 variant of β-casein, which appeared not to have the disadvantages of A1 β-casein.

The second part of this review is a critique of the A1/A2 hypothesis. For both DM-1 and CHD, the between-country correlation method is known to be unreliable and negated by recalculation with more countries and by prospective studies in individuals. The animal experiments with diabetes-prone rodents that supported the hypothesis about diabetes were not confirmed by larger, better standardized multicentre experiments. The single animal experiment supporting an A1 β-casein and CHD link was small, short, in an unsuitable animal model and had other design weaknesses.

The A1/A2 milk hypothesis was ingenious. If the scientific evidence had worked out it would have required huge adjustments in the world's dairy industries. This review concludes, however, that there is no convincing or even probable evidence that the A1 β-casein of cow milk has any adverse effect in humans.

This review has been independent of examination of evidence related to A1 and A2 milk by the Australian and New Zealand food standard and food safety authorities, which have not published the evidence they have examined and the analysis of it. They stated in 2003 that no relationship has been established between A1 or A2 milk and diabetes, CHD or other diseases." (Truswell, 2004)

Woodford devotes several pages in *Devil In The Milk* to answering Truswell's criticisms, and I think his effort is convincing. It is lengthy and in-depth ... I recommend that the reader go through it. Truswell chose to resort to a number of arguments which erroneously reported and interpreted data, were not even logical in places, and he did not present any convincing counter-evidence of his own. No conflicting data was offered.

His main three counter-arguments centered on (a) epidemiological studies and data do not establish proof, (b) that Elliott's prior mice and rat studies were invalidated by the larger, higher quality FAD trial, and (c) that rabbits were are inappopriate model for studying atherosclerosis. Well, we already know that correlation does not establish proof, and in fact, final proof is a very elusive element in science. As for the FAD trial, we know that it was seriously flawed and the conclusions invalid. About using rabbits as test animals?? ... it is a common, accepted model for a great deal of research of this type.

The tone of his paper is clearly negative, even resorting to the implication that the A1/A2 hypothesis was all an 'ingenious scheme'.

However, the axe that gives the final blow to Truswell's attempted expose' is that it was discovered later that he was under hire by Fonterra at the time ... Woodford's relentless and persistent investigation revealed that he was being employed by Fonterra as their 'key external scientific witness' in the 2004/2005 hearings with the New Zealand Intellectual Property Office, in which Fonterra ended up losing in all matters to A2

94

Corporation. Now this is truly an interesting scenario: Truswell was Fonterra's key witness in efforts to secure patents that would give them intellectual property rights and a marketing edge in *promoting* A2 milk (and the A1/A2 hypothesis) ... but then, after this legal battle was lost in full to A2 Corporation in the month of July, 2005, Truswell then went on to author a review attempting to trash the entire A1/A2 hypothesis four months later. The word 'trash' is appropriate in this respect ... both as the verb and then as the noun.

NZFSA update, October 10th, 2007

When *Devil In The Milk* was first published in New Zealand in September 2007 the response was immediate and extraordinare ... Woodford reports that he was interviewed through the radio and television media forty times in the first week. He explains that he heard nothing from Fonterra, except that they had contacted him just before publication, asking him to delay the publication for six months. The NZFSA, however "came out with all guns blazing".

The New Zealand Food Safety Authority published an update on October 10th, 2007 explaining that they were in communication with the European Food Safety Authority (EFSA) and confirmed that the EFSA was planning to review the possible health hazards of A1 β-casein-rich milk.

In the report, the NZFSA acknowledged Keith Woodford, and his book, *Devil In The Milk*, and the A1/A2 (BCM-7) hypothesis ... and also acknowledged the considerable media interest preceding and following the publication. The tentative NZFSA conclusion was:

> "There is no scientific consensus on this hypothesis and material presented in the book is open to scientific debate."

95

For this reason, their position regarding the A1/A2 issue was summed up by the Minister of Food Safety, Honorable Lianne Dalziel, in the following statement:

"I consider that as EFSA is undertaking a comprehensive review of the existing science associated with A1 and A2 milk, a separate New Zealand review, as originally proposed by NZFSA in October 2007, will not be necessary." (Dalziel, 2008)

The EFSA Report

The home page of the EFSA website states their purpose and scope as follows:

"The European Food Safety Authority (EFSA) is the keystone of European Union (EU) risk assessment regarding food and feed safety. In close collaboration with national authorities and in open consultation with its stakeholders, EFSA provides independent scientific advice and clear communication on existing and emerging risks."

(www.efsa.europa.eu/en/aboutefsa.htm)

The agency was established in January, 2002, with their head office in Parma, Italy. Their scope of responsibility extends to include animal health and welfare, and crop plant issues.

Their website goes on to say:

"EFSA's goal is to become globally recognized as the European reference body for risk assessment on food and feed safety, animal health and welfare, nutrition, plant protection and plant health. EFSA's independent scientific advice underpins the European food safety system. Thanks to this system, European consumers are among the best protected and best informed in the world as regards risks in the food chain."

96

This is heady wording! One cannot help but be impressed, and in fact, confident that with this agency we are going to receive a fair and responsible assessment.

The New Zealand Food Safety Authority (NZFSA) met with the EFSA in December, 2007, requesting that the EFSA review the A1/A2 milk (BCM-7) hypothesis. The EFSA accepted. It was clear that the NZFSA held the EFSA in high esteem, positioning them as a 'higher authority', which was stated in their April 2nd, 2008 report:

> "EFSA is a highly resourced, competent and internationally respected authority with a wealth of expertise in the areas of risk assessment and food safety."

With confirmation that the EFSA would undertake the review, the NZFSA once again concluded:

> "I consider that as EFSA is undertaking a comprehensive review of the existing science associated with A1 and A2 milk, a separate New Zealand review, as originally proposed by NZFSA in October, 2007, will not be necessary." (Dalziel, 2008)

The NZFSA worked with the EFSA, and made available all the data and studies which they had themselves acquired, specifically including the Swinburn report (this was mentioned in the DalZiel report)

The EFSA review is entitled *Review of the potential health impact of β-casomorphins and related peptides*, and is sub-titled a *Report of the DATEX Working Group on β-casomorphins.* The report was issued on January 29th, 2009. It took 13 months for them to complete the project, starting from when the New Zealand Food Safety Authority asked them to undertake the review in December, 2007. The report is 107 pages long. However, 39 pages are devoted to listing an impressive number of references ... 535 of them, in fact. This is more than impressive … it is many more than what I could find myself that are directly related to this issue … and there may be a reason for this. I will explain in the ensuing paragraphs.

An aside: the 'Betacasein.net' website, which is devoted to compiling up-to-date scientific literature on the A1/A2 issue listed only 80 studies in their 2008 review.

The conclusion to the report is contained in a two-sentence finale' at the end of their summary, and is curiously repeated as the totality of their 'Recommendations' at the very end of the report:

> *"Based on the present review of available scientific literature, a cause-effect relationship between the oral intake of BCM-7 or related peptides and aetiology or course of any suggested non-communicable diseases cannot be established. Consequently, a formal EFSA risk assessment of food-derived peptides is not recommended."*

This conclusion was probably predictable. Many, including Woodford, feel that it was. One has only to look at how the agency was tasked with the review, by whom, the studies specifically emphasized beforehand, and the conclusions already reached by NZFSA as a precedent. Perhaps much more importantly, however, the EFSA was faced with a horrendous problem if their conclusions favored the A1/A2 (BCM-7) hypothesis. For example, (a) it would send a panic message to the public not to consume A1 milk … that a potential health risk was involved; (b) it would turn the dairy industry totally upside down … telling them that they needed to convert the dairy herds, literally worldwide, to A2 producers … a process that would be incredibly expensive and would take as much as ten years or more to accomplish; (c) an immediate risk assessment and evaluation would be essential; (d) it would place a sudden and immediate burden on government and regulatory agencies to

98

inspect, monitor, and regulate; (e) it would require the creation of an extensive public awareness and information program, and (f) it would require labeling of milk and milk products to identify A1 and/or A2 content, including a statement of risk assessment.

Putting all this together, yes, it was predictable that they would choose a conclusion that would diffuse all these potential problems and responsibilities … in the hope that it would all 'blow away in the wind'.

What, who, is the DATEX Working Group ?

Now, who put this report together? The eight authors are identified as the 'DATEX Working Group on β-casomorphins', and are, as listed in the report: Ivano De Noni, Richard J. FitzGerald, Hannu J.T. Kornonen, Yves Le Roux, Chris T. Livesey, Inga Thorsdottir, Daniel Tome', and Renger Witkamp. Keith Woodford, once again the relentless investigator, concludes that five could be classed as dairy scientists with strengths in bio-chemistry, two were trained in veterinary faculties and now specialize in toxicology and pharmacology, and one is a nutritionist (Inga Thorsdottir, from Iceland). One cannot help but be a little skeptical about dairy scientists working on a study that could potentially turn their industry inside-out … and it may even be suggested that careers and job positions may be at stake. A veterinary background … ?? … with a specialty in toxicology and pharmacology … ?? … does this sound appropriate?

Interestingly, I. Thorsdottir is listed in the EFSA report's own references as the author or co-author of two studies related to the subject matter at hand, with, it turns out, very different conclusions from that of the report. After searching the literature, I found another two studies authored or co-authored by Thorsdottir, again involving research in the same field. I reviewed these studies in the previous chapter. All four studies strongly support the A1/A2 milk (BCM-7) hypothesis.

99

Another author was Ivano De Noni from Italy. My own research revealed that this author had also been involved in research which supported the A1/A2 milk (BCM-7) hypothesis. He was the sole author of a study published in the journal Food Chemistry in 2008 entitled *Release of β-casomorphins 5 and 7 during simulated gastro-intestinal digestion of bovine β-casein variants and milk-based infant formulas*. His finding was that the β-casomorphins 5 and 7 (BCM-5 and BCM-7) were released from only the A1 and B genetic variants of milk β-casein.

However, it seems that only Thorsdittor and De Noni had been involved in any previous studies concerning the A1/A2 (BCM-7) issue. And, amazingly, both of these author's prior studies reached conclusions supportive of the A1/A2 (BCM-7) hypothesis. As Woodford points out, where are the epidemiologists, the diabetes and heart disease specialists, the neurologists, or those who are specialists in food intolerance and leaky gut syndrome?

So, you ask: "How could these two authors, having been extensively involved with research supporting the A1/A2 milk (BCM-7) hypothesis, then agree with the conclusions of the EFSA report that directly contradicts their own conclusions from previous studies?" It is a good question!

One startling peculiarity of the study was that nowhere could I find a recommendation or an appeal for additional studies. Considering the over-all conclusion that the hypothesis is not proven, or is inconclusive, it would then make sense that additional study is desired. Via a quick run-through of the entire report I found 17 statements overtly implying that there was a need for additional research. Yet there was no direct appeal for further research, and the wording of the report seems to carefully avoid such an appeal. 'Recommendations' was listed in the table of contents as the very last section, and it was here that I hoped to find a recommendation for additional research. But instead, the 'Recommendation' contained only two sentences, which was a word-for-word repeat of the conclusion, (quoted above) saying nothing about the need for additional research. My own conclusion is that the 535 references were listed as a way of saying "no more study is necessary ... we already have 535 studies".

In addition, the study repeatedly stated that this or that was not *proven*, or that *cause and effect* was not established. For an exploratory study concerned primarily with risk assessment, this is very strange language. First, we know that absolute proof, especially proof of a *causal* relationship, is very elusive in scientific investigation. As I have pointed out, beginning in Chapter One and in the Appendix in the section entitled "An Intro to the Scientific Method, Research-Study Design, and Statistics", a bona-fide cause and effect relationship is almost never achieved in scientific investigation, and is not even insisted on as the primary goal. This is one reason we use statistical techniques ... to give us some sort of confidence that we are on the right track, and to give some sort of measure of our degree of success.

Secondly, one would assume that the EFSA is truly interested in *risk* as a first step ... after all, this is what they *say* is their main objective ... to assess risk ... so if potential *risk* is identified (not proof or certainty) then they should be the first to jump to attention.

There are a number of other grounds on which the report could be criticized ... but it is almost beside the point. The study and its conclusions were clearly pre-designed to placate the public and researchers by summing up the issue with 'there is no need for alarm', 'no risk assessment is warranted', and 'everyone can go on happily drinking their A1 milk without concern' ... and that the dairy industry can continue to produce it.

Sounds almost OK ... except for one small matter ... how about my and your health ? .... how about the health of our

101

babies and children ? .... and future generations ? ... and how about the increasing millions that suffer and *will* suffer from diabetes, heart disease, autism, schizophrenia, and other neurological disorders ? Should someone be perhaps thinking about *responsibility* ? Ugh !! .... what a nasty word !!

The Current Situation

It seems that the EFSA report has put many minds at ease, and, as with NZFSA, there is no pressure to make a risk assessment or to get excited about the potential health risk of consuming A1 milk.

Fonterra

Seven days after the EFSA report was released, the New Zealand 3-News network quoted Fonterra as saying the EFSA review on the safety of protein fragments in dairy products and other foods was in line with its own stance that different milks are safe to drink. None other than our well-known player, Jeremy Hill, now Fonterra's Group Director of Technology, concluded:

> "The review showed that different types of cow's milk are safe to drink and no one type of milk is safer than another." (3news, N.Z., February 5, 2009, 12:00 am)

One can only be amazed at how quickly and easily some scientists can jump the fence to protect their own personal interests.

U.S. Food and Drug Administration

Oddly, and a matter of concern for Americans, the U.S. Food and Drug Administration has not ventured any statement regarding this issue. A scrutiny of their website turns up zilch.

"What is going on?" you ask. Another good question. Woodford suggests that at the highest level in the American, Canadian, and European dairy industry, *and* within the various government regulatory and food safety agencies, the top executives are very aware of the issue, but are watching and waiting, hoping of course that it will all 'blow away in the wind'.

No call for additional research is being announced either. In fact, there has even been a recommendation that public funds should not be spent on further studies.

Fonterra, in the meantime, has been growing even larger, and expanding their marketing ever and ever wider, and becoming even more dominant as a dairy industry giant.

A2 Corporation has also been quietly increasing its footholds and trying to move into markets in other countries. They have succeeded in forming a couple of mergers with Australian companies, and have gained partial access to the Japanese market. However, their marketing attempt with Hy-Vee supermarkets in the U.S. was abandoned. And the proposal to market A2 milk in Korea under the 'Lotte' brand fell through. One apparent problem was that they could not guarantee the purity of their A2 milk … testing milk samples and preventing contamination by A1 milk is problematic. At the present time A2 milk is being marketed only in New Zealand and Australia. A2 Corporation reported a loss of $717,172 (Australian dollars) for the first half of 2010. (A2 Corp, 2010)

Even Dr. Woodford seems to have taken a rest on the A1/A2 issue, and all is relatively quiet. No new major studies have surfaced … the last one was the Russian Kost et al study mentioned above (2009), which showed an association between BCM-7 and a delay in psychomotor development in infants.

Concerning the situation in the dairy industry, Woodford reported the following to the International Farm Management Association at their 16th Conference, held in Ireland late 2007:

"INNOVATION FOR FUTURE PROFIT: Approximately 500 New Zealand (NZ) dairy farmers are converting their herds to eliminate production of A1 beta-casein within the milk. The alternative beta-casein is A2 beta-casein, and the associated milk is known as A2 milk. A2 milk can be considered the original milk before a mutation affected some antecedents of modern European breeds. A1 beta-casein and its derivative beta-casomorphin7 (BCM7) have been implicated in numerous health issues including Type 1 diabetes, heart disease and autism. There are now more than 100 relevant papers in peer reviewed journals. The broader NZ herd is also drifting away from A1 beta-casein production due to a serendipitous association between genetic merit as measured in NZ and A2 beta-casein. There is no evidence of this occurring in other countries. The farmer decisions can be structured using concepts of risk management and decision theory. However, analysis is complicated by uncertainty as to future premiums/discounts associated with A2/A1 milk. Outside of NZ most farmers know nothing about this issue."

Keith Woodford maintains a website entitled 'Posts from Keith Woodford' at www.keithwoodford.wordpress.com

Almost **all** *of the milk currently produced and sold in the United States is Type A1, or A1 contaminated.*

The *problem,* then, is two-fold. First, the discovery of the potential health hazard of drinking type A1 cow's milk challenges us to further investigate this potential and to take action to remove the risk. But a second problem emerges, and that is the refusal of the dairy industry to responsibly face the issue, and of our governments and government regulatory and food safety agencies' chosen 'head-buried-in-the-sand' posture. We are therefore first presented with strong evidence of a health risk factor, coupled secondly with the inability to do anything about it.

This situation is clearly unacceptable.

If the Type A1 (BCM-7) hypothesis is valid ... or even suspected of being valid ... then we have been deceived ... and continue to be deceived.

The importance of the statements at the beginning of this chapter thus become clear. It may not be so much a question of what science will eventually conclude ... although this is extremely important ... but may be more a matter of consumers knowing the truth, being protected, and having a choice. And what is at is at stake is not only a challenge to the dairy industry, but, much more importantly, is your and my health ... and the health of our babies and our children ... and of generations to come ... and the increasing millions who suffer and will suffer from diabetes, heart disease, and neurological disorders.

References For Chapter Three

3News, New Zealand, the article was entitled *Fonterra says EFSA review backs up its stance that milk is safe,* broadcast 12:00 am, Thursday, February 5th, 2009. A copy is available on their website at www.3news.co.nz/Fonterra

A2 Corporation; 2010 Mid-year Report, Available online from the A2 Corporation website

Dalziel, Honorable Lianne; Report to the New Zealand Office of the Minister for Food Safety, April 4th, 2008

European Food Safety Authority (EFSA); *Review of the potential health impact of β-casomorphins and related peptides,* Report of the DATEX Working Group on β-casomorphins, January 29th, 2009. Available online via the EFSA website.

New Zealand Food Safety Authority (NZFSA); *Beta casein A1 and A2 in milk and human health: Lay Summary,* Lay Summary to the Swinburn Report, Available online at www.nfsa.govt.nz/policy-law/projects/a1-a2milk/lay-summary.htm

Swinburn, B.; *Beta casein A1 and A2 in milk and human health, Report to New Zealand Food Safety Authority,* July 13th, 2004. Available online from the NZFSA website.

Truswell, A.S.; *The A2 milk case: a critical review,* European Journal of Clinical Nutrition, 2005; 59, 623-31

Truswell, A.S.; *Reply: The A2 milk case: a critical review,* European Journal of Clinical Nutrition, 2006; 60, 924-2

Woodford, K.; *An invited plenary paper to the International Diabetes Federation Western Pacific Congress, Wellington, 2 April, 2008.*

Woodford, K.B.; *A critique of Truswell's A2 milk review,* European Journal of Clinical Nutrition; 60(3): 437-39

Woodford, K.; *A2 Milk, Farmer Decisions, and Risk Management; Innovation For Future Profit;* A paper presented at the 16th Conference of the International Farm Management Association, held in Ireland, 2007

Chapter Four

IMPLICATIONS AND A CALL FOR ACCOUNTABILITY AND ACTION

We have a choice !

We can gullibly and passively submit to the profit motivated special interests of big business, the deplorable 'head-in-the-sand' complacency of our government food safety agencies, and stagnated science ....

Or, we can exercise our vote in both the political arena and in the marketplace to insist on responsible and courageous effort by those same parties to address this health hazard and to find and enact a corrective remedy.

AND, the identification of the BCM-7 peptide, the devil-in-the-milk, might very well be one of the most remarkable health discoveries of our time.   We suddenly have at our fingertips a potential key to eliminating a significant causal factor for chronic disease .... an opportunity to uplift our human health to a new and higher plateau !!

Implications

As suggested in the previous chapter, the challenge to the dairy industry and government regulatory and safety agencies could be monumental. An honest, responsible, and transparent approach to the Type A1 milk issue would unleash a number of reactions and required proactive steps:

1. It would send a panic message to the public not to consume Type A1 cow's milk … that a potential health risk was involved.

2. It would potentially turn the dairy industry totally upside down … telling them that they needed to convert the dairy herds, literally worldwide, to A2 producers … a process that would be incredibly expensive and would take as much as ten years to accomplish.

3. The scientific community would be prompted to seek alternative solutions.

4. An immediate risk assessment and evaluation would be mandatory.

5. It would place a sudden and immediate burden on government and regulatory agencies to inspect, monitor, and regulate.

6. It would require the creation of an extensive public awareness and information program.

7. It would require labeling of milk and milk products to identify Type A1 and/or Type A2 content, including a statement of risk assessment.

Dr. Keith Woodford is a farm management specialist, and has outlined the steps to be taken to convert existing dairy herds to non-Type A1 producers. He estimates that this process would take up to ten years. Conversion following his guidelines is already taking place in New Zealand, although it is helped inadvertently by the fact that almost all of the best dairy bulls in New Zealand happen to be Type A2 producers.

The conversion of dairy herds in the U.S., Canada, Europe, and other countries would require a concentrated and focused effort. It would be costly, both in terms of the actual conversion and also in terms of the lost market for Type A1 milk and the cost of measuring Type A1 content, regulation, monitoring, and labeling.

However, it could very well be that further scientific research and study could find a simpler solution. For example, infant formula manufacturers were prompted in the 70s and 80s to treat cow's milk-based formulas to decrease or eliminate the bioactivity of harmful peptides. More research may uncover a simple way to remove the BCM-7 *devil in the milk*, or render it harmless. Or, a simple and partial solution is to actively test and separate the milk variants at the farm and at the dairy. Even the Holstein-Friesian breed produces approximately 25% pure Type A2.

The Cloud May Have a Silver Lining

If one were to step back and view this situation from a much broader perspective, it may even be argued that we are overlooking a very strong *positive* aspect to this issue …. the identification of the BCM-7 casomorphin peptide might very well be one of the most remarkable health discoveries of our time … the knowledge of which we can use in a beneficial way.

We now know that a number of protein peptides are highly bioactive, and that a few of them can be very damaging to our bodily health. These peptides can be generated by several different proteins, both of plant and animal sources. They include grain gluten, soybean protein, animal meat protein, and milk protein. The two peptides which have thus far attracted the most attention is *gliadorphin*, from the gluten of wheat and *β-casomorphin* generated by the beta casein protein in Type A1 cow's milk. This situation has been with us for many generations.

So …. What do we do with these new discoveries ??

We can react negatively, pointing to the enormous implications to a major segment of our food industry, and complain that we are now being told to avoid yet another two common food substances, and take offense to what can be seen as an affront and a challenge to the 'proverbial goodness' of cereal grains and cow's milk. It is easy for us to react in this negative direction, and with what would seem to be good justification.

However, if we take a step back, and survey the situation in a broader and clearer perspective .... we can appreciate that what is really happening is that we suddenly have at our fingertips a key to eliminating a significant causal factor for chronic disease ... an opportunity and potential to uplift our human health to a new and even higher plateau !!

A Call For Action

We then come to the most critical crossroads of this entire expose. What do we do *now* ?? Do you, the reader, simply set this book and this new information aside and tell yourself "that this is all very interesting, *but* ...", or do you feel, as I do, that we must try to do something about it. We must be proactive and do something, even if just sending off an email or two, or discussing this with a friend, or asking your grocer if he or she knows about A1 milk and could you purchase A2 milk instead. Or maybe you could contact your government representative. Maybe even send off a protest to the FDA, the EFSA, or other government food safety authority. You could go even further and email known advocacy organizations. How about protesting to the dairy industry, even directly to the dairy farmers? Or even telling Walmart and Costco and Safeway that you want to have A2 milk available on the shelves, and refuse to buy A1 milk ...*and* you insist on appropriate labeling to let you know what you are spending your hard earned money on.

The option you choose is, of course, up to you. But by the time you have read this page, I, the author, will have sent a free e-copy of this expose to each and every U.S. senator and house representative, to each of the members of the U.S. House Committee on Agriculture and the U.S. Senate Committee on Agriculture, Nutrition & Forestry , to the FDA, EFSA, and other food safety government agencies, to over a hundred media contacts, to a number of advocacy organizations, to a host of milk and milk product processors, wholesalers, *and* retailers, to dairy organizations and co-ops, and finally to a large number of individual dairy farms.

I invite you to join me in this effort.

What is most important is that you simply add your voice in protest. It is the number of voices that is important ... I guarantee that if enough consumers demand A2 milk, it *will* be supplied, or if enough letters are send to our government representatives, they *will* respond, and the same can be said for all the other players. Your emails can be very brief ... as little as 50 words ... or you can expand, as you see fit.

To assist in this endeavor, the following is a collection of contacts which I have gathered together to get the ball rolling, so to speak. If you are completely lost for words, you are welcome to use the suggested wording that I have included for each type of contact.

1. Your government representatives

a. For members of the US House of Representatives, you can go to www.house.gov/ and "write your representative". You will be led to a pathway where you can identify your representative for your district and to a contact form.

My suggested email text is as follows:

Dear ……

I am sending you this email because I am deeply concerned about the Type A1 milk issue and the BCM-7 peptide which this variant of cow's milk can produce. I

111

am aware of the health risk to myself and my family by drinking Type A1 milk. I am also aware that almost all milk currently sold in the U.S. contains Type A1 milk. Further, I understand that the FDA, the EFSA, and other government food safety agencies know about this issue but have never-the-less taken a 'head-in-the-sand" stance. Plus, there is no program being actively pursued to promote further research, nor to prompt the dairy industry to convert their dairy herds to A2-only producers, or to pursue other ways to help correct this malady.

I therefore ask you as my representative to actively support investigation into this issue. I would like to have Type A2 milk available at my local grocery outlet, with proper labeling to insure that I know which variant of milk I am purchasing.

Sincerely, _____

b. The second contact would be the U.S. House Committee on Agriculture, which can be accessed by the same link, or go directly to AgRepublicanPress@mail.house.gov I suggest the same text, except to modify it slightly to indicate that you are addressing a committee instead of a single representative.

c. Next, you can contact your U.S. senator by linking to www.senate.gov and go to "Contact My Senators". The same text as above would again be appropriate.

d. The U.S. Senate Committee on Agriculture, Nutrition & Forestry can be contacted by using their website at www.agriculture.senate.gov/ Again the above suggested text can be used as a guideline.

If you live in the UK, similar contacts can be accessed via the link www.parliament.uk

In Canada, the link is www.canada.gc.ca

For Australia, the link is simply Australia.gov.au

2. Contacting government food safety agencies

a. On March 14th, 2009, the Obama administration formed a special food safety organization named *The Food Safety Working Group*, which may be especially appropriate to address our advocacy effort. Their website and email contact is www.foodsafetyworkinggroup.gov/ContentContactUs/HomeCon tactUs.html

b. The Canadian government has a similar government organization, *The Canadian On Farm Food Safety Working Group*. Their website is www.onfarmfoodsafety.ca and the suggested email address is karen@cfafca.ca

c. Another U.S. government sponsored food safety agency is *The Center for Food Safety and Applied Nutrition*, with two email addresses given: industry@fda.gov & consumer@fda.gov

d. A high level U.S. organization is *The Office of Disease Prevention and Health Promotion*, with a website at www.odphp.dhhs.gov They have a contact form at www.hhs.gov/accessiblityassist.html

e. *The European Food Safety Authority* (EFSA) has become the recognized international leader in matters concerning food safety, as discussed in Chapter Three. This is then the most important government food safety organization to send a protesting email. Their readily accessible website is at www.efsa.europa.eu which will then lead you to "ask EFSA service". Clicking on that will give you some options, and at this point it seems that they really don't what to hear your protest. However, if you choose the "staff directory" instead, you can get into their organization a bit deeper. You again have a number of options where to go. I suggest you choose the "Risk Assessment Dictorate" and email the Director of Risk Assessment, which is Riitta Maijala, and her email is Ritta.Maijala@efsa.europa.eu You may feel that contacting another staff member or another

113

EFSA department is more appropriate ... I leave the choice up to you.

I feel that the EFSA warrants special treatment, and I suggest the following text:

Dear Ritta Maijala, Director of Risk Assessment,
European Food Safety Authority

I am forwarding this email because I am deeply concerned about the Type A1/A2 milk issue and the BCM-7 peptide which the A1 variant can produce. I am familiar with two books on the subject, *Devil In The Milk*, written by Dr. Keith Woodford, and *Don't Drink A1 Milk* by Brent Bateman. The research and scientific studies presented in both these expose's is compelling and credible, and concludes that consuming Type A1 milk (and the BCM-7 peptide) presents a potential for serious health risk to myself and my loved ones.

I am aware of the EFSA January 29th, 2009 report entitiled *Review of the potential health impact of β-casomorphins and related peptides*, in which the EFSA concluded that a formal risk assessment is not recommended. After reviewing what Woodford and Bateman have written, and as a concerned consumer, I strongly feel that something is very much amiss here. As Bateman states in his book, what goes beyond the scientific debate is that consumers are told the truth, are protected, and have a choice. And I feel he is correct is saying that what is at stake is my health, and that of my babies, and of generations to come.

If there is truly a connection between the BCM-7 peptide and such illnesses as diabetes, heart disease, and neurological disorders ... even a small one ... then we are genuinely at risk of increasing the harm caused by

114

these diseases, and we are being deceived by our governments and the dairy industry.

I therefore implore your agency to review the evidence and your report, to promote and support additional research, and to act courageously with transparency and integrity to remedy this issue. Simply put, I would like to be able to purchase A2 milk at my local grocery, and avoid the A1 variety, and I insist on appropriate labeling to insure that I know which variant I am feeding myself and my family

           Sincerely,   _____.

f. For Americans the U.S. Food and Drug Administration (FDA) is also a key contact choice. Their website is at www.fda.gov and the link for consumer questions and comment is consumer@fda.gov

Again I feel that the wording for this agency may need to be thought through. I suggest:

Dear U.S. Food and Drug Administration (FDA)

I am forwarding this email because as a consumer I am deeply concerned about the Type A1/A2 milk issue and the BCM-7 peptide which the A1 variant can produce. I am familiar with two books on the subject, *Devil In The Milk*, written by Dr. Keith Woodford, and *Don't Drink A1 Milk* by Brent Bateman. The research and scientific studies presented in both these expose's is compelling and credible, and concludes that consuming Type A1 milk (and the BCM-7 peptide) presents a potential for serious health risk to myself and my loved ones. I have viewed your website, but I do not find anything that is related to this issue. I am aware of the EFSA January 29th, 2009 report entitiled *Review of the potential health impact of β-casomorphins and related peptides*, in which the EFSA concluded that a formal risk assessment is not

115

recommended.   After reviewing what Woodford and Bateman have written, and as a concerned consumer, I strongly feel that something is very much amiss here. As Bateman states in his book, what goes beyond the scientific debate is that consumers are told the truth, are protected, and have a choice. And I feel he is correct is saying that what is at stake is my health, that of my babies, and of generations to come. If there is truly a connection between the BCM-7 peptide and such illnesses as diabetes, heart disease, and neurological disorders ... even a small one ... then we are genuinely at risk of continuing and even increasing the harm to fellow Americans caused by these diseases, *and* we are being deceived by our governments and the dairy industry. I therefore implore your agency to investigate this issue.   Simply put, I would like to be able to purchase A2 milk at my local grocery, and avoid the A1 variety, and I insist on appropriate labeling to insure that I know which variant I am feeding myself and my family. I fully intend to exercise my vote in both the political arena and in the marketplace to promote A2 milk and discourage the A1 variety.

           Sincerely,   _____.

Britain has its own food safety and food standards agency, the Food Standards Agency. Email contact can be sent via www.food.gov.uk or directly to helpline@foodstandards.gsi.gov.uk

Canada also has their own food safety agency, named simply Food Safety, with a website at   www.foodsafety.gc.ca   The website is a little confusing and it is not clear where we should direct our protest. However, it would be prudent to send your email to the Chief Public Health Officer, Public Health Agency of Canada. A contact form is available for this purpose at the website.

The New Zealand Food Safety Authority (NZFSA) can be accessed at   www.foodsafety.govt.nz and enquiries are directed to nzfsa.info@maf.govt.nz

The NZFSA has previously acted as a bi-national agency for both New Zealand and Australia. However, New South Wales now has its own food safety authority (NSW Food Authority) and has recently taken over much of the food safety duties for the   whole   of   Australia.   Their   website   is   found   at www.foodauthority.new.gov.au   and   email   is   directed   to contact@foodauthority.nsw.gov.au

3. Advocacy organizations

There are a large number of advocacy organizations out there, and I cannot pretend to be an expert in this respect, nor is my list anywhere near complete, but here are a few that seem suitable for us. The text message can be short and to the point. Here is my suggested text:

Dear Sir/Madam …

I am writing this email to you in order to place my support for initiatives directed to the dairy industry, the various government food safety agencies, and to government representatives, to take action to remove the health hazard associated with the consumption of Type A1 cow's milk and the BCM-7 peptide that it can generate.

I would like to refer you to the evidence presented in the book written by Dr. Keith Woodford, *Devil In The Milk,* and the expose' by Brent Bateman entitled *Don't Drink A1 Milk.* I strongly feel that the evidence is compelling and credible, and that the potential risk to our health cannot be ignored. I agree with Bateman's statement that what is at stake goes beyond the scientific debate … we are dealing with the issue of consumer awareness, consumer protection, and having a choice.

117

If there is truly a connection between the BCM-7 peptide and such illnesses as diabetes, heart disease, and neurological disorders ... even a small one ... then we are genuinely at risk of increasing the harm caused by these diseases, and we are being deceived by our governments and the dairy industry. As a consumer and a care-giver for my loved ones, I encourage more research on this issue, and programs put in place to correct the health hazard. I would like to have Type A2 milk available on my grocer's shelves, with proper labeling to ensure that I know which variant of milk I am purchasing.

I therefore request that you apply your talents and efforts as a consumer advocate to help in the fight to remove this health hazard.

Sincerely, _____

NP Action (S.T.O.P. Safe Tables Our Priority)
npaction@npaction.org

Keep Our Food Safe
www.keepourfoodsafe.org (email form on website)

US PIRG
www.uspirg (contact form on website)

Consumer Federation of America
www.consumerfed.org   Email: cfa@consumerfed.org

Center for Science in the Public Interest
www.cspinet.org   Email: cspi@cspinet.org

Safe Food International
www.safefoodinterntional.org   Email:sfi@cspinet.org

National Farmers Union
www.nfu.org (contact form on website)

Union of Concerned Scientists
www.ucsusa.org   (contact form on website)

Marne Rowland Duke
www.linkedin.com/in/marneduke   (contact form on website)

Food and Water Watch
www.foodandwaterwatch.org   (contact form on website)

Mindfully.org
www.mindfully.org   (contact form on website)

Food Secure Canada
www.foodsecurecanada.org   (contact form on website)

Food Safety News
www.foodsafetynews.com/contact-us

Center for Foodborne Illnesses Research & Prevention
www.foodborneillness.org Email: cfi@foodborneillness.org

The Center for Food Safety
www.centerforfoodsafety.org
Email: office@centerforfoodsafety.org

Food Quality news.com
www.foodqualitynews.com   (feedback form on website)

Public Citizen
www.citizen.org   (contact form on website)

4. Grocery Retailers and Wholesalers

Next, we can target the marketplace, and let our grocery retailers and wholesalers know that we are aware of the Type A1/A2 issue and that we want to be able to purchase only Type A2 milk. This is where we, the consumers, have the ultimate power and the final say. I can assure you ... if we, the consumers, refuse to buy A1 milk and place our vote in the marketplace for A2 milk only, then the suppliers and the dairy

119

industry as a whole *will* bow to our demands! It is a guiding principle of our economic system.

An important part of our message to this group is to demand appropriate package labeling to ensure that we know that we are buying Type A2 milk, and have some sort of assurance of the purity. This is an important issue on its own, because much debate has already taken place with other milk concerns ... whether or not the milk being purchased comes from cows that have or have not been treated with rBGH, for example.

I have a list of 49 of some of the largest retailers and wholesalers. The list is by no means comprehensive or in any sense complete, but it pretty well covers the major global suppliers, with an emphasis on the market in the U.S. and Canada. Trying to find an appropriate contact is sometimes difficult when searching these websites, and there are often a number of different options. I encourage the reader to be innovative and to explore contacts other than what I have listed. You may wish to try to contact a senior executive directly, for example. It is of course up to you.

I am starting with HyVee Supermarkets, because they *did* have Type A2 milk available on their shelves during the years 2006 and 2007, supplied to them by the Australian-based A2 Corporation. It is not clear what the reason was that they finally discontinued marketing A2 milk in 2008, but it is suspected that a problem emerged with guaranteeing that the milk was not contaminated at least in part with A1 milk. If there is not a lot of support in the dairy industry, it becomes a logistic and testing nightmare to ensure that the milk being sold is pure A2. We can, however, encourage HyVee to try again.

Hy Vee Supermarkets
   www.hy-vee.com/company/contact/

A suggested text for our message to Hy Vee could be as follows:

Dear Hy Vee Supermarkets:

I am sending this email to encourage you to try making Type A2 cow's milk available once again on your shelves.

I am very aware of the Type A1/A2 (and BCM-7 peptide) issue and I feel very strongly that I would like to protect myself and my loved ones from the potential health hazard associated with consuming Type A1 milk.

I sincerely thank you for your efforts in this respect, and I look forward to seeing A2 milk available in your outlets once more.

Sincerely, _____

For all the other companies, the suggested text could be modified as follows:

Dear _____:

I am sending you this email to encourage your company to make Type A2 cow's milk available on your shelves.

If you are unaware of the distinction between types A1 and A2 cow's milk, and the potential health hazard associated with consuming Type A1, I refer you to *Devil In The Milk*, written by Dr. Keith Woodford, and *Don't Drink A1 Milk*, by Brent Bateman. Type A1 cow's milk is genetically different from Type A2 in that it can generate the BCM-7 peptide, which has been found to be causally linked with diabetes, heart disease, and neurological disorders.

I feel that the evidence is credible and compelling, and cannot be ignored, although our dairy industry *and* our government food safety agencies have chosen a 'head-in-the-sand' approach on the issue. It seems that they do not want us to know about this issue. As a consumer and a care giver, however, I choose to do my best to protect

121

myself and my loved ones from the potential health hazard linked to consuming Type A1 cow's milk or milk products using Type A1. I therefore request that your company investigate this matter and somehow make Type A2-only milk available, with appropriate labeling to ensure that I know that I am buying A2 milk.

Sincerely, and thank you for your attention to this issue,

Walmart   We all know about Walmart!
   www.walmartstores.com/contactus/feedback.aspx#3

Carrefour   French based, very large internationally
   Gerald Diot, Gerald_diot@carrefour.com
   Phillippe Bovani, phillippe_bovani@carrefour.com
   Sylvain Ferry, sylvain_ferry@carrefour.com

Ahold   Large Netherlands based chain
   www.ahold.com/contact

Metro Group   German based, known for Future Store concept
   www.metrogroup.ro/internet/site/metrogroup/node/10122
   (contact form on website)

TESCO   U.K. based, huge internationally
   www.tesco.com/help/contact/contactus4.asp

KROGER   U.K. based, very large internationally
   www.kroger.com   (customer comments form on website)

SEVEN&I Holdings Co. Ltd.   Japan based, owner of 7-Eleven
   www.webdairy.7-eleven.com:7001/CR/General_Request.jsp
   (contact form on website)

REWE Group   German company, over 11,000 stores world-wide   www.rewe-group.com/en/kontakt

Target   U.K. based, world-wide outlets
   www.target.com/gp/help/display-contactus-form

COSTCO   Over 450 stores in seven countries
   www.costco.egain.net/system/selfservice.controller
                  (contact form on website)

AEON   Japan based, purchased Carrefour in that country
   info@aeonfood.com/56129/inquiry

CASINO GROUPE   France based, 9,000 stores in 15
   countries   www.groupecasino.com/en/Presse-Relations
      (contact form on website)

AUCHAN   France based, has expanded into Russia,   China,
   and Morocco
      www.auchan.fr/components/pageFooter/formQuestion

INTERMARCHE   France based, also in Spain and Germany
   www.intermarche-seyssins.com/livraison-domicile
      (contact form on website)

LIDL   German chain, discount stores customer.service@lidl.ie

ALDI   German chain of discount stores
   www.everesthosted.com/aldi/feedback/Concern.asp

ALBERTSONS   Second-largest supermarket chain in U.S
   www.shopalbertsons.com/ContactUsAction.do

EDEKA   German company, also in Eastern Europe
   info@edeka.de or   presse@edeka.de

SAFEWAY   U.S. company, U.S. and western Canada
   www.safeway.com/IFL/Grocery/Comments

E. LECLERIC   French company, partner with CONAD
   www.e-leclerc.com/afdetail.asp   (contact form on website)

SPAR   Based in Netherlands, largest retailer in world
   info@spar-international.com

TENGELMANN   German company, very large, own A&P in U.S.   www.foodbasics.ca/en/contact

J SAINSBURY PLC   Large U.K. based chain
www.sainsbury.co.uk/contacts

MORRISONS   Large U.K. chain
www.morrisons.co.uk/store-finder/about-customer

DELHAIZE GROUP   Belgium company, large in U.S.
www.delhaizegroup.com/en/Contacts
media@delhaizegroup.com

KMART   Australia based company, also in N.Z. and U.S.
www.kmart.com.au/ContactUs/FeedbackForm.aspx

WOOLWORTHS   Largest supermarket chain in Australia
www.woolworthslimited.com.au   (contact form on website)

LCL   Loblaw's is Canada's leading retailer chain
Customer_Service@loblaw.ca

SUPERVALU   U.S. chain with 900 stores in 19 states
www.supervalu.com   (contact form on website)

PUBLIX   U.S. chain mostly in southern states
www.publix.com/contact/ContactUs.do

FOOD LION   U.S. arm of Delhaize, owns Sweetbay and
Bloom outlets   www.foodlion.com/CustomerService/Email

C&S WHOLESALE GROCERS   Second   largest   food
wholesaler in U.S.   helpdesk@cswg.com

MEIJER   U.S. chain, mostly in eastern states
www.custhelp.meijer.com/app/ask

H-E-B   Large chain in Texas, Louisiana, and Mexico
www.heb.com/contact-us/Contact-us.jsp

A&P   U.S. and Canada chain, owned by Tengelmann
apcustomerrel@aptea.com

WINN DIXIE   U.S. chain
www.winndixie.com/contact_US/contact_US.asp

SOBEYS   Canada's second largest chain
www.sobeyscorporate.com/en/Contact-Us.aspx

DOLLAR GENERAL   U.S. chain with 7,500 stores in 30 states
www.dollargeneral.com/OurStoresPages/CustomerService.aspx

BJ'S WHOLESALE CLUB   U.S. chain, owner of Big Box
www.bjs.com/contact-us.content.contact_us.A.about

GIANT EAGLE   U.S. chain
www.gianteagle.com/contact-us

METRO INC   Canadian chain in Quebec and Ontario
www.metro.ca/on/utilities/contact.en.html

AWG   U.S. chain   contactawg@awginc.com

ROUNDYS   U.S. chain, mostly in Wisconsin
Robert Mariano, CEO/Chairman   rmariano@roundys.com

PATHMARK   U.S. chain, based in New Jersey
www.pathmark.com/contactUs.asp

NASH FINCH COMPANY   U.S. based wholesaler, serves US military   www.nashfinch.com/contact.cfm

WHOLE FOODS MARKET   U.S. based, world's largest retailer of natural foods
www.wholefoodsmarket.com/company/service.php
(contact form on website)

STATER BROTHERS   U.S. chain, based in California
www.staterbros.com/Top-Menu/Contact_Us.asp

5. Contacting the Media

The best media contact is your local newspaper. Try to contact an editor direct, especially the editor of a feature section that deals with food, nutrition, or related topics. I have found that it is not easy to create any excitement or even a response from media folks, but it is certainly worth a try. You may have to use a little 'newsroom' type language to catch their attention.

A letter to the editor is usually in the 200 -300 word range, and the following is a suggested text (200 words):

Dear Editor:

What has happened with the recent and startling discovery that the Type A1 milk we buy in our supermarkets can generate a highly disruptive peptide called BCM-7, which is causally linked with diabetes, heart disease, and neurological disorders? The New Zealand farm management specialist, Dr. Keith Woodford, explained the evidence and warned us of the health risk in *Devil In The Milk*, and a new book by a nutritionist, Brent Bateman, *Don't Drink A1 Milk,* reveals that the dairy industry and government food safety agencies are deceiving us and have chosen a 'head-in-the-sand' approach, even discouraging further research. I feel that he evidence is credible, compelling, and cannot be ignored. There is an urgent need for you and I, the consuming public, to place our vote in both the political arena and the marketplace to correct this deception and wrongly directed complacency. The message is *not* to drink Type A1 cow's milk, and to insist on properly labeled Type A2 only.

If you feel you can get away with a little bit longer text, you can use (400 words):

Dear Editor:

And so, I ask … what has happened with the recent and startling discovery that the Type A1 milk we buy in our supermarkets can generate a highly disruptive peptide called BCM-7, which is causally linked with diabetes, heart disease, and neurological disorders? The New Zealand farm management specialist, Dr. Keith Woodford, explained the evidence and warned us of the health risk in *Devil In The Milk*, and a new book by a nutritionist, Brent Bateman, *Don't Drink A1 Milk,* reveals that the dairy industry and government food safety agencies have chosen a 'head-in-the-sand' approach, even discouraging further research … they do not want us to know about this issue. Their stance is perhaps understandable, due to the enormous implications … but their complacency is wrongly directed.

I cannot help but conclude that some mischief is at play. We, the forever malleable consumers, are once again being deceived. I feel that the evidence is credible, compelling, and cannot be ignored.

And why, I ask, do we hear nothing about this issue from the FDA or other food safety agencies, nothing from the U.S., Canadian, or European dairy industry, and the safer Type A2 milk is *not* available on our grocer's shelves … yet New Zealanders and Australians *can* buy A2 milk in *their* stores, and New Zealand dairy farmers are quietly converting their herds to Type A2-only producers.

As a concerned consumer, and a health provider to my family and loved ones, I (a) refuse to purchase Type A1 cow's milk or its products, (b) encourage dairy farmers and retailers to provide and properly label Type A2 milk, and (c) demand that our government and the dairy

127

industry as a whole play a more proactive role to eliminate the health risk of A1 milk.

From a more positive perspective, we may have at our very fingertips a key to eliminating a significant cause of chronic disease and a chance to uplift our human health to an even higher level.

Sincerely, _____

If you care to try a more formal approach, there is an excellent site at www.theopedproject.org that lists over one hundred U.S. newspapers that have both a 'letter to the editor' link and an 'op-ed' link. The op-ed, or 'opinion to the editor' format allows for text in the 600 -1200 word range, but requires that the text be more formal and substantive. Please refer to the website if you need more information. Remember to include your name, address, and contact information. Almost all editors request that you do not send attachments. I would suggest the following text for the op-ed option:

Dear Editor:

The 2009 report by the European Food Safety Authority (EFSA), entitled *Review of the potential health impact of β-casomorphins and related peptides*, attempted to extinguish potential public concern about the health hazard of consuming Type A1 cow's milk. It seems that it was successful in its mission. Few people in the U.S., Canada, and Europe have even heard about the distinction between the genetic variants of cow's milk, broadly divided into Type A1 and Type A2 ... and even less about the highly bioactive BCM-7 peptide that Type A1 can generate, and especially its causal link with diabetes, heart disease, and neurological disorders. No one is demanding A2 milk, no one is voicing concern about the harmful effects of the BCM-7 peptide, and there is no program among American, Canadian, or

128

European dairy farmers to convert their herds to Type A2-only producers. Further research has been discouraged ... no one is seeking a way to neutralize the bioactivity of the BCM-7 peptide, or to find new ways to modify A1 production in favor of A2.

However, it is a somewhat different story in Australia and especially New Zealand, where the bulk of the scientific studies originated. Due to the efforts of one company, the A2 Corporation, A2 cow's milk is available on the shelves of N.Z. and Australian grocers, and New Zealand dairy farmers are quietly converting their herds to A2-only producers. Dr. Keith Woodford, a New Zealand farm management specialist, studiously and carefully outlines the evidence and warns us of the health risk in *Devil In The Milk*, and a new book by a nutritionist, Brent Bateman, *Don't Drink A1 Milk,* reveals that the dairy industry and government food safety agencies have chosen a 'head-in-the-sand' approach, even discouraging further research. Together they demonstrate that the evidence of the bodily harm that the BCM-7 peptide can do is credible, compelling, and cannot be ignored. Plus they reveal that the EFSA review is seriously flawed.

One cannot help but conclude that some mischief is at play. We, the forever malleable consumers, are once again being deceived. Once again big business and their government cohorts are attempting to hide the truth and suppress the facts underlying an urgent health issue. The EFSA has said nothing since the January 29th, 2009 report. The FDA has been completely silent on the issue. There is no program among U.S., Canadian, and European dairy farmers to convert their herds. No retailers or wholesalers are attempting to procure and market A2 milk.

129

It may not be so much a question of what science eventually concludes, although this is of course extremely important, but it may be even more a matter of you and I, the consuming public, being made aware, being protected, and having a choice.

There is a critical need for you and I, concerned consumers and health providers for our families and loved ones, to place our votes in both the political arena and the marketplace to correct this deplorable misdirection and unwarranted complacency, to (a) refuse to purchase Type A1 cow's milk or its products, (b) encourage dairy farmers and retailers to provide and properly label Type A2 milk, and (c) demand that our government and the dairy industry as a whole play a more proactive role to eliminate the health risk of A1 milk.

However, *the cloud may have a silver lining:* from a more positive perspective, we may have at our very fingertips a key to eliminating a significant cause of chronic disease and a chance to uplift our human health to an even higher level. Our governments, our dairy industry, and you and I, the consuming public, urgently need to act with courage, integrity and transparency to resolve this health issue and to move on to improved human health.

Sincerely, _____

The following is a shortened list of newspapers that are more national or international, rather than addressing only their immediate locality. I have also added a few popular national news magazines.

Wall Street Journal
Op-Eds: 600-1200 words, double-spaced. E-mail edit.features@wsj.com

Letters: 300-word limit. Send comments to Timothy Lemmer (letters editor) at wsj.ltrs@wsj.com

USA Today

Op-Eds: 600-800 words. Fact-based approach. Include background information--qualifications for writing about subject, basic contact information. E-mail the Forum Page Editor at theforum@usatoday.com (No attachments).

Letters: Letters of 250 or fewer words have the best chance of being published. Submit online at asp.usatoday.com/marketing/feedback/feedback-online.aspx?type=18 or e-mail editor@usatoday.com

New York Times

Op-Eds: Suggested length is 750 words. Refer to http://www.nytimes.com/2004/02/01/opinion/and-now-a-word-from-op-ed.html?pagewanted=2 for tips and email address.

Letters: 150 words or less. Send e-mails to: oped@nytimes.com.

Los Angeles Times

Op-Eds: 750 words average. Send to oped@latimes.com

Letters: Fill out form at http://www.latimes.com/news/opinion/la-comment-oped-cf,0,2007619.customform. Typically 150 words or less. May also email directly at letters@latimes.com

Washington Post

Op-Eds: Advised 800 words or less. The best way to submit article is using the online form at http://projects.washingtonpost.com/opeds/submit/.

Letters: Submit by e-mail letters@washpost.com

Daily News (New York, NY)

Op-Eds: 550 words or less. E-mail: nobrien@edit.nydailynews.com

Letters: Submit by e-mail to voicers@edit.nydailynews.com

New York Post (New York, NY)
Op-Eds: E-mail: cunningham@nypost.com
Letters: Submit online at http://www.nypost.com/sendletter,
or send to letters@nypost.com

Chicago Tribune (IL)
Op-Eds: 500-600 words. Email is preferred method of
submission ctc-comment@tribune.com
Letters: Submit by e-mail: ctc-TribLetter@Tribune.com, or
online http://www.chicagotribune.com/news/opinion/chi-
lettertotheeditor,0,3578487.customform.

Newsday (Long Island, NY)
Op-Eds: 700-800 words. Submit as open text
to oped@newsday.com
Letters: 250 words or less. Email letters to the editor
at letters@newsday.com

The Christian Science Monitor
Submissions: Preferably 750 or less. The Op-Ed page invites a
written version of what you might imagine the conversation
would be like at a cozy dinner party with interesting people:
serious, funny, broad-ranging discussion . The Op-Ed editor is
Josh Burek. More info
at http://www.csmonitor.com/About/Contributor-
guidelines#international

Boston Globe (MA)
Op-Eds: 700 words preferred. Email to oped@globe.com or
clicking on link
at http://www.bostonglobe.com/news/opeds/opeds.aspx?id=6524
.

Letters: Limit 200 words. Submit via online form
at http://www.bostonglobe.com/news/opeds/letter.aspx?id=6340
or email to letters@globe.com

The Commercial Appeal (Memphis, TN)

Op-Eds: 800 word limit. Use same e-mail or web form as letters to the editor.
Letters: E-mail letters@commercialappeal.com or submit onlineat http://www.commercialappeal.com/letter-to-editor/.

Boston Herald (MA)
Op-Eds: 650-800 words. E-mail: oped@bostonherald.com
Letters: E-mail to: Letterstoeditor@bostonherald.com

The Advocate (Baton Rouge, Louisiana)
Letters: Submit via online form
at http://www.2theadvocate.com/help/letters.

San Francisco Chronicle (CA)

Op-Eds: "Open Forum" 550 words or fewer.
Email forum@sfchronicle.com with subject title "For Open Forum."
Letters: 200 words or less. E-mail
toletters@sfchronicle.com

Contra Costa Times (East Bay area of CA)
Op-Eds: E-mail 650 words or less to clopez1@cctimes.com .
Letters: Letters must be 200 words or fewer. Email
to ccnletters@bayareanewsgroup.com

Miami Herald (FL)
Op-Eds: Under 650 words for weekly editions of the paper. Send by e-mail to oped@MiamiHerald.com . Include a head-shot.
Letters: Submit via online form
at http://www.miamiherald.com/contact-us/ or email
to HeraldEd@MiamiHerald.com

The Record (Bergen County, NJ)
Op-Eds: 800 words or less. E-mail: **oped@northjersey.com**
Letters: E-mail: letterstotheeditor@northjersey.com

The Hartford Courant (CT)

Letters: E-mail: letters@courant.com or submissions may be filled out at the following web form: courant.com/about/custom/thc/thc-letters,0,86431.customform.

Austin American-Statesman (TX)

Letters: Submit via online form http://www.statesman.com/opinion/content/feedback/letters ubmit.html.

News & Observer (Raleigh, NC)

Letters: 200 word limit. Submit via online form at http://www.newsobserver.com/about/newsroom/editor/.

Boston Herald (MA)

Op-Eds: 650-800 words. E-mail: oped@bostonherald.com
Letters: E-mail to: Letterstoeditor@bostonherald.com

Daily News (Los Angeles)

Op-Ed: 600-700 words. E-mail to dnopinion@dailynews.com
Letters: 100 words or less. Submit via online form at: http://www.dailynews.com/opinions#letter_form, or e-mail to dnforum@dailynews.com
Opinionated Q&A: Each week, readers are asked to weigh in on a particular topic. E-mail responses to opinionated@dailynews.com .

The Globe and Mail (Toronto, ON Canada)

Instructions are: If you're sending your letter or article by e-mail, the contents must be sent in the body of the e-mail message as plain text only. Please do not use Microsoft Word format or rich text format (RTF), and please don't send the letter or article as an attachment.

Comment Submissions: The Comment Editor at G &M is Natasha Hassan who can be pitched to at nhassan@globeandmail.com .

Letter: Should be less than 200 words. Submit to letters@globeandmail.ca .

The Root (published by Washingtonpost.Newsweek Interactive)
Essays: Should be 500-800 words in length. Please copy and paste the essay within the body of the email, as well as attach it as a Word document. Please send submissions, along with a one paragraph author bio, and phone and email contact information, to submissions@theroot.com .

AOL News

Op-Eds: The recently launched Opinion section of AOL news is a forum for discussion and debate on the top news of the day. The opinion editor there, John Merline, is actively looking for good opinion pieces that are fact and reporting based and will appeal to a general audience. Preferred length 600-650 words. Ccheck out Sphere.com and visit their Opinion tab. You can also contact Mr. Merline at john.merline@corp.aol.com .

The Nation
Submissions: Only accept e-mail queries for freelance submissions . Paste query (250 words briefly summarizing the issues, your conclusions, and your expertise on the matter) into the form located at: http://www.thenation.com/contact/smis
Letters: No longer than 300 words (the shorter the letter is, the more likely that it will be published). Please include a postal address and phone number. For the print edition, submit your letters here: http://www.thenation.com/contact/lett For online publication, submit your letter to: http://www.thenation.com/contact/webletter

Time Magazine
This is heady … but why not! An 'email the editor' from is available at
www.secure.customersvc.com/wes/servlet/CustomerService/

Newsweek

You can send a letter to the editor at: letters@newsweek.com. If you feel up to it, you can also try to publish an essay in the feature section 'My Turn' ... send your essay to myturn@newsweek.com

US News & World Report

Send a letter to the editor using the contact form at www.usnews.com/usnews/usinfo/infomain.html

6. Talking to the farmers

And last, but certainly not least, we need to carry our protest to the dairy industry itself, especially the farmers, to first of all make them aware of the Type A1/A2 issue, and then to encourage them to take remedial action. Below is a short list of a few of the main U.S. dairy farm organizations, co-ops, and breeders. A complete list for the U.S., and especially if we include the international scope, would be huge. I will leave it to your discretion to add additional contacts. By the time you have read this, I will have sent a free e-copy of my book and an attached letter to these contacts plus as many of the 110,000 dairy farms in the U.S. as I can find contacts for. Yes, the U.S. alone maintains 9.2 million dairy cows on a total of more than 110 *thousand* farms ... mostly small family-owned farms combined in co-ops and larger marketing units.

My suggested test for a proposed letter would read as follows:

Dear ....

I am writing to you as a concerned consumer and health care provider in regards to the Type A1/A2 milk issue and the potential health hazard created by exposure to the BCM-7 milk peptide, which can be generated from Type A1 cow's milk.

I first of all would like to make sure you are aware of the scientific basis for the issue, and then I hope to encourage you, as a key player in the dairy industry, to be proactive and to work courageously and with integrity to remedy this very serious dilemma.

I refer you to the scholarly book written by the New Zealand farm management specialist, Dr. Keith Woodford, *Devil In The Milk*, in which he studiously explains first the science in support of the issue, and then the mischievous and political haggling which has led to the suppression of the facts and a very successful effort by the dairy industry and government food safety agencies to placate the public. A follow-up to Dr. Woodford's work is a new expose' by a nutritionist, Brent Bateman, which adds to Woodford's work and reveals that the January 29th, 2009 report by the European Food Safety Authority (EFSA) entitled *Review of the potential health impact of β-casomorphins and related peptides* is seriously flawed and that the EFSA, the NZFSA, the FDA, and other government food safety agencies, in cohort with the dairy industry, have chosen a 'head-in-the-sand' stance.

We now know that there are at least fifteen different genetic variations of the 209 amino-acid chain of beta-casein milk protein, broadly divided into Type A1 and Type A2, depending on whether or not there is a *proline* amino acid or a *histidine* amino acid at position 67 of the chain. The proline is known to be the original, 'normal' configuration, and that the replacement by a histidine amino acid at that location was the result of a mutation several thousand years ago in the Holstein-Friesian breed. The histidine at position 67 was discovered first, and thus all variations with this configuration are considered to be A1. Those with the normal proline at position 67 are considered to be A2.

In-depth research over several decades revealed that, upon digestion in the human intestine, the beta amino

137

acid chain would bend just before position 67 if there was a histidine present at that point, and a seven-amino-acid chain would easily separate and break off. This fragment, or peptide, has become known as the highly disruptive BCM-7 peptide, Dr. Woodford's *devil in the milk*. More research, and a long process of 'putting the pieces of the puzzle together' revealed that the BCM-7 peptide can initiate harmful autoimmune reactions, is a strong oxidant, and a powerful opiate. It can attach itself to the insulin-producing beta cells in the pancreas, prompting an autoimmune response that can destroy the beta cells, thereby leading to diabetes. The BCM-7 molecule can oxidize LDL cholesterol, contributing to the build-up of plague in the arteries, or atherosclerosis. It is can also pass through the *blood-brain barrier* and act as an opiate, creating havoc with normal brain function, promoting neurological disorders such as schizophrenia and autism.

Most of the research, and the playing out of the intrigue and mischief which followed, took place in New Zealand … the story reads like an adventure saga. Interestingly, much of the research originated within the New Zealand dairy industry itself, notably with the New Zealand Dairy Board prior to its replacement by Fonterra when the New Zealand government privatized much of its industry in 2001. During that early period the N.Z. Dairy Board and Fonterra were very supportive of the A1/A2 (BCM-7) hypothesis, and actively sought to acquire copyrights to marketing A2 milk. A farm program to convert dairy herds to A2-only producers was also started. One of the scientists involved in the research and a noted New Zealand entrepreneur formed a company named the 'A2 Corporation', which competed with Fonterra for the copyrights. In the year 2005 the New Zealand government ruled in favor of A2 Corporation in all matters pertaining to the A2 copyrights, and thus the stage was set for Fonterra to reverse its stance on the issue and to become a powerful force to undermine and suppress the A1/A (BCM-7) hypothesis. They were very successful, and found that they had the support of the New Zealand Food Safety Authority (NZFSA) and eventually that of the EFSA as well.

Their support may be easy to understand ... the proposition that Type A1 milk presents a health risk carries with it an enormous implication. Almost all of our milk on the market is either A1 or contaminated with A1. And the Holstein-Friesian is, as you know, the most popular and the highest producing of all breeds. A1 and A2 milks are mixed at both the farm and at the dairy ... to test and separate them would constitute a logistic nightmare. Marketing a new A2 milk would involve a vast marketing expenditure. And what about the A1 that suddenly no one would want to buy? Even Dr. Woodford's prescribed procedure to convert dairy herds to A2-only producers would require a focused effort over at least a ten-year period. The government food safety agencies would be faced with problems as well. They would be required to make a genuine and honest risk assessment. More research would need to be encouraged, and funding made available. The public would need to be warned, and informed. Testing and monitoring would become a requirement. As would appropriate labeling. Standards would have to be decided on, and a way derived to enforce them.

So it is easy to understand why the dairy industry *and* the NZFSA, EFSA, FDA *and* governments in general would prefer that all of us common folk just didn't know about this issue, or that we be placated by a high-sounding report by a big name 'authority', with the hope that it will simply all 'blow away in the wind'.

But a lot of us may be reluctant to swallow all of this, especially without question. For one thing, what is at stake is our very health, and the health of our babies, and of generations to come. And what about those who suffer, and *will* suffer, from diabetes, heart disease, and neurological disorders? What may be even more important than what science eventually concludes, although this has a high priority, is that the consumers are told the truth, are protected, and have a choice.

While American, Canadian, and European consumers *and* farmers, know little, if anything, about this issue, and A2 milk is not made available on our grocer's shelves, and there are no farm programs or initiatives to breed out A1 production or even to separate the two varieties, the situation in New Zealand and Australia is quite different. Through the efforts of A2 Corporation A2 milk *is* available in the down-under supermarkets, and the New Zealand dairy farmers are quietly converting their herds to A2-only producers. There is an additional irony: the humped cattle common to Asia, the Nordic breed in Iceland, and the Normande breed in France are all almost pure A2 producers. Dairy farmers in the U.S., Canada, and most of Europe may one day wake up to find that that their A1 milk cannot be sold, while A2 milk from other countries is garnishing the market.

Our human history is a long continuous saga of obstacles being met and overcome … this is not even a big one. And there may very well be a *silver lining* to it all … on the positive side, we hold at our very finger tips a key to eliminating a significant cause of chronic disease and an opportunity to uplift our human health to an even higher level.

I therefore urge you, as a part of the dairy industry, to act proactively, with courage and integrity, to help us eliminate this dreadful malady, and to create a healthier world.

Sincerely _____

You can, of course, send a much shorter note to simply add your voice to the crusade. I will be sending a letter similar to the one above to as many farmers as I can. A few dairy contacts are:

Dairy Farmers of America
Their website is www.dfamilk.com, and email contact can be kdale@dfamilk.com or webmail@dfamilk

Holstein Association USA
A contact form is available at www.holsteinusa.com

Holstein World
The website is at www.holsteinworld.com and a comment can be placed on their website blog at kjohnson@dairybusiness.com

Dairy Farm International Holdings Ltd
A contact form is available at www.dairyfarmgroup.com

The Global Cow, Ltd.
You can contact Julie at Julie@globalcow.com, and their website is at www.globalcow.com

The Cattle Site
A contact form is on their website at www.thecattlesite.com

Mayfield Dairy Farms
Is one of the largest farms and also a co-op. A contact form is available on their website at www.mayfielddairy.com

Al Safi Dairy Company
Would you believe that the largest dairy farms in the world are in the Middle East? This one is in Saudi Arabia, and can be

141

emailed at info@alfaisaliah.com, and their website is at www.alfaisaliah.com

Fair Oaks Farms
A very nice website at fofarms.com, and can be emailed at info@fofarms.com

Arla Foods
Is a major milk processor and wholesaler, with a website at www.arlafoods.ca or www.arlafoods.com A contact form is on the website.

Robert Wiseman Dairies
Their website is at www.wiseman-dairies.co.uk and they can be contacted by email at care@wiseman-dairies.co.uk

Dairy Crest
Is another United Kingdom giant, with a website at www.dairycrest.co.uk and can be emailed at consumercare@dairycrest.co.uk

Almarai Dairy Farm
Their website is at www.almarai.com, with a contact form available.

Grupo Lala
Can be emailed at customerservice@lalafoods.com, with a website at www.lalafoods.com

Huishan Dairy
China now has several giant dairies as well. Huishan Dairy has a website at www.huishandairy.com

Stew Leonard's
Is a very large U.S. dairy wholesaler. A contact form is available on their website at www.stewleonards.com

Indian Farmers Fertilizer Co-operative, IFFCO
A contact form is on their website at www.iffco.com

HauXia Dairy Farm
Another Chinese giant farm, with a website at www.huaxiadairyfarm.com and an email address at info@huaxiadairyfarm.com

Bettencourt Dairy
You can email them at dairyoffice@bettencourtdairy.com and their website is at www.bettencourtdairy.com

Threemile Canyon Farms, LLC
They have a contact form on their website at www.threemilecanyonfarms.com

Crafar Farms
Their website is www.crafarms.co.nz and their email address is info@crafarms.co.nz

Food Retail World
One of the largest dairy retailers, with a website at www.foodretailworld.com. A contact form is available onsite.

APPENDIX

A. An Intro to the Scientific Method, Research-Study Design, and Statistics

One way to try to understand the world around us is via simple empirical observation and the application of the techniques of the *scientific method*. This may seem obvious and not even worthy of discussion, but misunderstanding what the scientific method is all about can lead to some seriously wrong assumptions and conclusions. The subject matter of this treatise is a good example.

The basis of all scientific inquiry is 'observation'. We observe phenomenon and then form a theory, or hypothesis, to explain the phenomenon, which we then attempt to 'prove'. In biological science the 'proof' usually means that we have established a true 'cause-and-effect' relationship.

However, we know from the start of any scientific study that a true cause-and-effect relationship and 'proof' of a theory or hypothesis is very elusive. You may have heard such statements as "proof is never established", or "cause and effect are never known", or "correlation does not imply causation", or "a hypothesis is always a hypothesis". A favorite of mine is "you cannot make a valid conclusion until all the evidence is in" … and in science all the evidence is never in … such is the nature of science investigation. Take the theory of gravity as a simple example: I'm sure that you feel confident each time you pick up a stone and release it from your fingers that it will fall to the ground. In your life you have done this, or something similar, countless times. In your mind 'gravity' is far more than just a theory ... it is a proven fact! Yet, in the strict scientific sense, it still remains just a hypothesis. It *may* be possible that just once that stone will *not* fall to the ground. And now you read of such a thing as 'anti-gravity' ... so maybe gravity is just a theory after all.

So we set aside true 'cause-and-effect' and 'proof' as goals which we know even before we start are unlikely to be reached, and we settle for lower level goals and ways to somehow let us know we are on the right track, and to measure our degree of success. This becomes particularly necessary in the biological sciences, because things happen at such a miniscule scale and often very quickly, so that we are obliged to 'observe at a distance' and to estimate what is happening based on results in the larger organism, rather than viewing the actual process first-hand. As a compromise to saying "this causes that", we say that "this is *associated* with that". If we feel more confident about the perceived association, we might call it a *relationship*, or even a *linkage*. But our scientist peers admonish us very quickly if we were to claim cause-and-effect, or proof.

To give a research study more of a sense of validity, then, we try to select a methodology, or study design, that gives us the highest credibility, and we employ the wonderful techniques of *statistics* to measure such things as incidence, prevalence, correlation, 'strength of association', degree of confidence, probability, and predictability. We are also confronted with a number of obstacles which we must try to avoid or overcome. These include *bias* or non-objectivity, limited or inaccurate data, false assumptions, illogical conclusions, and the presence of confounders. All of these concerns come to play in the analysis of the A1/A2 milk and BCM-7 issue.

As stated, all scientific investigation is based on empirical observation. However, the types of studies can be further separated into purely observational studies, clinical studies, and intervention studies. When studying humans and animals,

145

purely observational studies usually involve the observation of a population, or some segment of that population, and can be retroactive, current, or prospective (going into the future).

Population studies are referred to as *epidemiological studies* and terms used to describe the outcome include *incidence, prevalence,* and *correlation.* Incidence is simply the number of those in the population with the targeted disease or condition, prevalence is the *percentage* of the population with the condition, and correlation refers to the comparison of the incidence or prevalence of at least one factor which is thought to be a possible cause of the targeted disease or condition, with the incidence or prevalence of that targeted condition. The great disadvantage of epidemiological studies is that establishing cause-and-effect is even more distantly removed than with other study designs ... especially because potential *confounders* can render the entire study useless. A confounder is a separate factor from that being analyzed which can also explain the correlation or outcome. For example, we saw in the study of Type A1 and A2 milk that the correlation of the consumption of A1 milk in Finland with the incidence and prevalence of diabetes and heart disease is very high, but the high prevalence of these two disease conditions *might* be caused by a totally different factor, such as high saturated fat consumption, or alcohol intake, or a combination of other factors. The investigator, of course, will address and discuss potential confounders in his study, if he is being thorough and honest.

This brings us to the problem of *bias.* Bias, or non-objectivity, can be non-intentional, or it can be intentional. Non-intentional bias can be the result of poor study design, or simply the awareness of the investigator or subject about what is going on and their subsequent involuntary influence to affect the outcome. This type of bias can also be thought of in the very broad sense as a product of the investigator's or subject's world view, or paradigm. Directly to the point, this could be a pro-bias in the study of the pros and cons of drinking cow's milk due to the inner belief by the investigator or subject in the proverbial goodness of milk ... an outcome of over a hundred years of advertising by the dairy industry and the teachings of mom and the school teacher. Now *that* is a difficult bias to overcome!

With the A1/A2 milk issue we saw that intentional bias can also be at play, with the FAD Trial, the Truswell study, and the reviews by the New Zealand Food Safety Authority and the European Food Safety Authority, as examples.

A great deal of effort is normally undertaken by the investigating scientist to negate bias. One of the most lauded techniques is to design the study so that it is *randomized* and/or *blinded*, or *double-blinded*. By randomized we mean that the subjects are selected 'randomly', no one knowing beforehand which subjects are selected. By blinded we mean that the subject does not know which treatment is being administered or double-blinded when both the subject *and* investigator do not know which treatment is used.

It is important to note, especially in the context of the studies done in support of the A1/A2 (BCM-7) hypothesis, that epidemiological studies, particularly when surveying entire populations, are naturally *randomized* and *blinded* ... the entire population is the subject group, and the question of whether the subjects or investigator can influence the outcome is mute ... it is simply a matter of collecting data.

With clinical studies we apply laboratory techniques to study phenomena in greater detail, and in which we can control inputs. Such studies can be simply laboratory analysis, or can be controlled trials, such as with animal models. Animal models were used in some of the studies of the A1 milk, BCM-7 hypothesis. Animal models can be very useful, but are often derided as not being the same as using humans, and the choice of animal may be critical. The rat, mouse, and rabbit are common choices, depending on what is being studied. The use of animals for clinical trials has become a very exacting science of its own,

147

with the animals being bred for particular traits that are being targeted. This is particularly true for diabetes and heart disease.

The other broad category of scientific studies are human intervention studies, where the subjects being studied are given different treatments and then studied. The time element can be current, or longitudinal … going back in time, or 'retrospective', and/or going ahead in time … 'prospective' The goal is to narrow down the type of intervention to the one which most closely determines or predicts the targeted outcome.

B. ABOUT THE SERIES

The Nutrition Factor:

A Bold New Perspective

Overview

I have undertaken this series for the purpose of offering nutrition information to the general public. I feel I have much to offer, and I perceive a great need for the public to be correctly informed about the subject of their nutrition. During the years that I have studied nutrition I have been dismayed by popularist styles of writing which for the most part either attempt to sensationalize one single concept or nutrient, or, frankly, present erroneous information. I have been equally dismayed by the failure of nutrition scientists, the professional nutritionist community, and the medical profession to attempt to communicate with integrity and transparency directly to the public.

The series begins with the introduction of two basic concepts. The first is the notion that, contrary to the conventional wisdom in nutrition, *it is very difficult to obtain all of our required nutrients from simply "eating a variety of basic foods and maintaining a balanced diet".* The implications of this new perspective are enormous and far-reaching.

The second basic concept is that *our food supply has changed dramatically over time, and our physiologies were designed during an ancient era; these two factors combine to question the adequacy and suitability of our modern food choices and eating habits.*

The two concepts make up Part One and Part Two of the series, and with Part Three I discuss a host of nutrition concepts and research findings. Together, the three parts present *A Bold New Perspective.*

One central issue in understanding the new perspective, and the need for it to be presented, is the exposure and analysis of the conventional wisdom in nutrition and medical practice and science … which can be described as the prevailing nutrition and medical science "paradigm". I suggest that the existing paradigm is not only erroneous, but that it is leading us in a very wrong direction in health care and our understanding of the factors influencing individual health .

About the Paradigm

The Problem of Individual, Group, and Cultural Bias

The notion that scientific inquiry can be subject to bias and misinformation by the influence of strongly held points of view, doctrines, and/or beliefs by the researchers is a surprise to most people not familiar with scientific study, and also to many of those who *are* involved, even the scientists themselves. This was especially true in earlier times, when science and medicine were held in great esteem and their territory thought to be hallowed. This reverence suffered a great challenge when it became clear that science was subject to major shifts in direction, and that sacred tenets held to be absolute by one generation crumbled when critically scrutinized by another.

149

Probably the foremost thinker in this new way of viewing the progress of science was Thomas S. Kuhn, author of *The Copernican Revolution* (1957, 1985) and *The Structure of Scientific Revolutions* (1962, 1970, 1996). His central observation was that the progress of science jumped in revolutionary steps, in almost a generation to generation fashion, with an earlier generation of scientists dogmatically pursuing one singular pathway, or paradigm, unswayed until a newly arrived generation challenged that pathway and was able to move on to a new perspective, a new paradigm.

Thomas Kuhns' insights have become generally known and appreciated among academics, yet his observation still holds. In more recent times it has been suggested that we no longer jump from one paradigm to a totally new one, but instead we experience a *paradigm shift*. Whether it is a shift or a jump to a whole new paradigm is a matter of debate.

Nowhere is the existence of a paradigm more clear than in modern medicine, and nutrition, as taught and practiced in Europe, the United States, and other Western countries.

So .... how can this paradigm be described ... and what is wrong with it ... and how should it be changed ... or *shifted* ??

Nutrition is *Not* a Part of Mainstream Medicine

One characteristic of the prevailing paradigm in mainstream medical science is the reluctance to take the subject of nutrition seriously. When you or I think about bodily health, we quickly include nutrition as a key factor ... it is common sense ... yet your practicing medical doctor is not nearly so agreeable to do the same. Yes, he will eagerly discuss nutrition ... from the perspective of diet ... but *not* as a bona-fide part of medicine itself. Yes, he will recognize the disease conditions caused by outright deficiencies of essential nutrients, but more of a concession rather than an acceptance ... and he will stubbornly refuse to consider possible health benefits of additional nutrient intake beyond that needed to prevent the deficiency diseases, such as scurvy, caused by a deficiency of vitamin C, or rickets caused by very low intakes of calcium.

This failure to include nutrition as an integral part of the core of medical science can be illustrated by the dismal failure to teach nutrition to pre-med and medical school students. As an example, the University of Hawaii is a standard, fully accredited American university, with the attached John Burns School of Medicine, and the usual accredited undergraduate curriculums in pre-med, nursing, medical technology ... and nutrition and food science as well ... the FSHN Department where I earned my Bachelor's of Science degree in human nutrition. My nutrition curriculum was essentially the same as the pre-med curriculum, with the same courses in biology and zoology and physiology, general chemistry and organic chemistry, and biochemistry. Except that I was required to study more biochemistry and a host of specific nutrition classes. Much of my class time was therefore with pre-med students, and in study-group and study-hall sessions as well. The pre-med students were my classmates. I admired them greatly, for they were the smartest of the smart, dedicated to their studies, and intensely focused. Whenever I entered a new class at the beginning of a semester, and saw that many in the class were pre-meds, I groaned, knowing that getting an "A" in this class was going to be tough.

I noticed even from the beginning courses that the pre-med students had little interest in nutrition, per se. Yes, they would diligently study in the areas that 'brushed' alongside nutrition ... in physiology, biology, and biochemistry, but they did not delve deeper, and they were diffident to entering discussions with me about the subject of nutrition. Perhaps they were so focused on their immediate studies that they had no time to explore what was considered a non-essential subject ... or perhaps they were already attuned to omitting nutrition as a bona-fide part of medicine. No nutrition courses were required by the pre-meds at

151

UH, although the nursing students were obligated to take one course in their final semester. I audited that course, and knew it well, and was surprised to observe that the nursing students were reluctant to study nutrition as well. Why, I wondered at the time.

The pre-med and medical school curriculums are standardized and follow accreditation guidelines, but they are not *required* to teach nutrition. Neither does the American Medical Association require nutrition education, and knowledge of nutrition is *not* required to get through medical internship and finally become a practicing medical doctor.

The Failure to Teach Nutrition in Pre-Med and Medical School Curriculums

Searching for some statistics about nutritional education in medical schools, I came across an excellent study by Frank M. Torti, et al, which reported the results of a survey taken July 1999 to May 2000 of 122 U.S. medical and osteopathic medical schools (which is just about all of them ... I understand there are a total of 125). (Torti et al, 2001) Of the 122 schools, 98 responded, with 95 providing detailed information. Of these 95, one indicated outright that they did not offer nutrition education, and 94 claimed to offer nutrition education. Of these 94 schools, 32 did not specify how their required nutrition was taught, 25 stated that nutrition was integrated into other courses, only 31 had stand-alone nutrition courses, and 6 had strictly optional nutrition education, which included library or independent study. This, then, indicated that 88 schools claimed to offer some nutrition education.

Within these 88 schools, the courses in which nutrition was taught were designated as follows: Nutrition, 31; Biochemistry, 7; Physiology, 3; Integrated curriculum, 11; and Clinical practice, 4. In other words, only 31 had courses that included 'nutrition' in the title or description.

Even more revealing, however, is the reported number of hours of instruction in nutrition by each of the 88 schools. Twenty-five of the schools reported giving equal-to-or-less than 10 hours of instruction, 37 schools reported 11 – 20 hours, 17 gave 21 – 30 hours, 3 gave 31 – 40 hours, and *only 5 schools gave greater than 40 hours of nutrition education.*

At this point, I would like to say this: studying biochemistry or other biology courses in a medical curriculum is *not* the same as studying nutrition … believe me, I know. For example, I took the 440-441 courses in biochemistry taught to the pre-med students at UH, and I also studied biochemistry as taught within our FSHN curriculum … they are definitely *not* the same. And, even 40 hours of instruction is really nothing … the beginning Nutrition 101 alone provides over 50 hours of in-class instruction.

And so, where and how does a typical medical physician learn what they know about nutrition ?? I suggest that they receive their knowledge from the same sources that you do … from the news of the day and from popular magazines, and from books found for sale at Barnes & Noble, Borders, or other popular book stores. Yes, it is true that they are better equipped to understand and interpret nutritional information, with their background in the biology sciences and chemistry, but it is only a matter of degree. While good textbooks in nutrition *are* available, they are not commonly so … I have noticed that your typical bookstores do not stock good nutrition textbooks, especially for advanced nutrition, and I doubt that many physicians bother to take a trip to the university bookstore to actively search for good nutrition textbooks.

Then Why Are Medical Doctors Considered To Be The Authority On Nutrition ??

So, then, why are medical doctors thought to be experts on nutrition?

153

Throughout my years of studying nutrition I have tried to understand this reluctance by the medical community to give nutrition its due priority status. I must admit that the answer is not fully clear to me, even now, but I do have some insights. One clue comes from studying the history of medicine and nutrition.

Walter Gratzer, in his fascinating review of the history of nutrition, in *Terrors of the Table,* (2005) explains that the roots of Western medicine, and nutrition, goes back to Hippocrates of Cos (fifth century BC), whose theory was based on the concept of the *four humors*. The four humors were thought to be bodily counterparts to the four elements: earth, air, fire, and water. The teachings of Hippocrates was later reinforced by Galen of Pergamum, named "The Prince of Physicians" (second century AD), whose doctrines were considered immutable for 15 centuries. Much can be said to explain this early view of medicine, which also included a theory of nutrition, but one central tenet of the Galen paradigm was that disease and ill-health was caused by factors from *outside* the body, not by malfunctions *within* ones physiology. When considering food (and its nutrients), Galen taught that poor health resulted from *excesses*, rather than deficiencies. For example, Gratzer reports that Galen bragged that his father had lived to 100 because he avoided eating fruit his entire life … fruits were given the attributes of 'cold' and 'moist' and thought to cause diarrhea and fevers. It is amazing that this belief predominated for so many centuries … probably contributing to much of the malnutrition and infant mortality during those times.

A historical example of how the doctrines of Hippocrates and Galen influenced nutrition is the case of vitamin C.

The deficiency disease condition caused by an insufficient intake of this essential nutrient is 'scurvy', which can be a truly hideous disease. In early Scotland it was called "blacklegs" because of bloody patches forming under the skin. It can cause

154

rotting of the gums and loss of teeth ... and hair. A sufferer may characterize extreme lassitude, or constipation so persistent that surgery may be required, and the victim often emits an intolerable stench of putrefaction.

It is curious that only a very few species in the entire animal kingdom cannot produce their own vitamin C ... humans are one of this select group. Others in the group include the chimpanzee, the gorilla, the guinea pig, the fruit bat, and one species of birds. Each of these species are supplied with ample vitamin C in their normal environment, suggesting that somewhere in our humanoid ancestral history we too lived in an environment with ample vitamin C and thus lost our ability to produce our own. Humans lack the liver enzyme *gulonolactone-oxidase*, required to catalyze the last step in the metabolic pathway to produce vitamin C. Your dog and cat, the horse, the cow, the elephant ... all can produce their own vitamin C ... but you cannot.

The saga of vitamin C is long and filled with historical intrigue, starting from when scurvy was first identified as a specific disease condition in the time of Hippocrates, and even before, until vitamin C was finally isolated as ascorbic acid ... white crystals derived from lemons, oranges, paprika, cabbage, and adrenal glands ... accomplished in the years 1928-31. Scurvy was often a major factor in the outcome of historical battles and epic voyages of exploration. It was an issue with the Crusaders of the Middle Ages. During Vasco da Gama's voyage to the Indies half of his crew died from scurvy. A four-year circumnavigation by the Commodore Anson started with seven ships and 2,000 men and ended with only 600 men surviving ... 4 had been killed in battle, the rest were lost to scurvy. A report on the effect of the disease among British sailors during the 1700's concluded that 19 deaths in every 20 had been the result of scurvy (John Hammond, 1747). Scurvy has been reported as a major cause of death in countless historical scenarios: the Mormons making their way to Utah in the mid 1800's, the siege of Paris in 1870, the siege of Kut-el-Amara in 1916, during The Great War (WWI), among the prospectors during the California gold rush, and during episodes of war and famine even today.

We all know that vitamin C, or ascorbic acid, is readily available from fruits and vegetables. An intake of only 16 milligrams per day is enough to ward off the ravishes of scurvy. We know that scurvy is the result of a deficiency ... it is the inability of the body to function because it lacks a nutrient .. *not* because of a virus, or an infectious attack from outside the body, or an excess intake of some substance. Yet it was the insistence that scurvy was caused by such external factors that prevailed for many long centuries, retarding the discovery of its cure and blocking the knowledge of the foods that could be eaten to prevent it. Galen's theory of humors, supported by the high prevalence of scurvy among sailors, concluded that the condition was caused by 'bad air' ... the damp air of the oceans or within the dark bilges of ships ... or by the excess intake of salt. The notion that consuming citrus fruits could prevent scurvy was unthinkable ... according to Galen doctrine, citrus fruit was "the commonest cause of fevers and obstructions of the vital organs".

Gratzer writes that one of the earliest challenges to the prevailing wisdom of the time was a book entitled *The Chirurgeon's Mate*, written by John Woodall in 1617. He had advocated eating fruits as a cure for scurvy, but he and his theory was paid little heed. One hundred and thirty years later, in 1747, a British naval surgeon named James Lind performed a clinical trial aboard the HMS Salisbury which illustrated the value of citrus fruits in preventing scurvy, but by the time of his death in 1794 he and the results of his study were all but forgotten. Captain Cook, and several physicians who followed his thinking at the time, thought they had found a cure with 'sweetwort' in the 1770's. But it wasn't until a Scottish naval doctor named Gilbert Blane advocated the intake of lime juice that scurvy finally became controllable. Blane had seen the results of scurvy while serving with the British navy in the Carribean during the war with France in the 1780's. During one 12 month period 60 seamen had died in battle in the Carribean ... over 1600 from scurvy. Through his efforts scurvy was almost absent among the British navy by the beginning of the 19th century. Laboratory work done by Harriette Chick and her team in 1918 and published in the medical journal, *The Lancet*, finally put all debate to rest, and it became accepted that something in limes prevented scurvy. It was the end of a 300 year struggle against an entrenched paradigm. Ten years later ascorbic acid was isolated and identified as the 'vitamin' in limes that could prevent scurvy.

What is truly amazing in all of this is how one paradigm, filled with such error and misinformation, could prevail over the minds of intelligent men and women so completely and for so long. It is a lesson to consider. And when one looks critically at the reluctance of today's medical community to 'look within' for explanations and cures of disease conditions ... the intake of essential nutrients, for example ... then one cannot help but conclude that today's medical science is suffering from a hangover of a previous, long-antiquidated paradigm.

How often have you heard a medical doctor explain that this or this condition, the actual cause unknown, is probably due to a virus or infection from an outside source? How often have you heard it explained that the condition is not because of a nutrient deficiency, but by *too much* of a nutrient, or an excessive intake of one substance or another? Could this thinking be a ghost of a paradigm from a distant past?

This is a complete aside, and perhaps I should be scolded for stating it, but the Galen paradigm's preoccupation with outside factors and causes rather than looking within is paralleled by the prevailing religious doctrine of the same period. I am, of course, talking about Christianity. It is to be noted that while some religions such as Buddism and Hinduism teach that we seek

157

knowledge, and salvation, from within, Christianity teaches that we seek knowledge and our salvation from outside sources. Plus the notion that our physiologies and God-given food supply is 'perfect', and therefore cannot be considered the source of ill health.

The emphasis of seeking explanations and cures for disease conditions and ill-health from *outside*, and in turn choosing to subordinate or ignore influences that take place *within*, such as with metabolism of nutrients, then, is one characteristic of the prevailing medical science paradigm.

It is prudent, however, to recognize and pay tribute to the tremendous success that medical science has had in identifying and eradicating infectious disease and diseases that truly *do* have an outside source. This cannot be understated. The progress and success, especially in the past two centuries, has uplifted our human health, increased our longevity, and eradicated a long list of diseases.

At the same time, however, a re-appraisal of the conventional wisdom is long over-due ... it is time for a *paradigm shift*.

In summary, the conclusions of *The Nutrition Factor: A Bold New Perspective* include (a) that there is a need to re-appraise our conventional wisdom regarding nutrition, (b) that medical science and the health care community need to give more attention and support to the study of nutrition, (c) that nutrition needs to be instated as a bona-fide and central part of medicine itself, and (d) that we need to critically examine the nature and characteristics of our modern food supply and its compatibility with our physiologies.

The implications are far-reaching and enormous. New research needs to be encouraged ... research that is objective, carried out with integrity and transparency, and with the researchers bravely accepting new challenges. We need to investigate the potential for improving the nutritional value of our foods and to adjust our food choices and eating habits in order to obtain better nutrition. The medical schools and pre-med curriculums need to be revised to include advanced study in nutrition, and nutrition needs to be a required subject of study.

C. A Rare Inspirational Insight

Before entering the UH undergraduate program in Food Science and Human Nutrition, I sought to 'test the waters' by auditing the one nutrition course that was required by the 4-year nursing students, as I mentioned above. Our instructor was a rare lady, indeed. She was from the faculty of the associated John Burns Medical School, yet she had an extensive background in nutrition. During the semester she often referred to her experience working in the field of international nutrition in several developing countries. On the first day of class ... and I will never forget this ... she approached from the front, holding her hands high and using her fingers to simulate quotation marks, and made a wonderful statement. It was a statement that was an inspiration to me at the time, and continues to be an inspiration even now. It also sums up the 'bold new perspective' of this series in a single phrase.

Later, as student editor of the FSHN Newsletter, I ventured to ask her permission to quote her inspirational statement. She was horrified: "No, you cannot do that ... they would kick me out of the medical school !!"

What she had said, in that memorable moment, went like this: "Why nutrition ?" she asked, with her fingers high and fluttering, "Because we now know that, at least in the United States, *long term health care is nutrition* !!"

159

References For The Appendix

Eaton, B.S.; Shostak, M.; Konner, M.; *The Paleolithic Prescription,* Harper & Row Publishers, 1988

Gratzer, W.; *Terrors of the Table: The Curious History of Nutrition,* Oxford University Press, 2005

Harris, M.; *Good to Eat, Riddles of Food and Culture,* Waveland Press, Inc. 1985, revised 1998

Johnson, F.E.; *Nutritional Anthropology*, Alan R. Liss, Ince, 1987

Kuhn, T.S.; *The Copernican Revolution, Planetary Astronomy in the Development of Western Thought,* Harvard University Press, 1957, 1985

Kuhn, T.S; *The Structure of Scientific Revolutions,* University of Chicago Press, 1962, 1970, 1996

Torti, Frank M. Jr.; Adams, Kelly M. MPH, RD; Edwards, Lloyd J., PhD; Lindell, Karen C., MS, RD; Zeissel, Steven H., MD, PhD; *Survery of Nutrition Education in U.S. Medical Schools – An Instructor-Based Analysis*, Medical Eduction Online, Vol. 6, 2001, Department of Nutrition, University of North Carolina at Chapel Hill, Medical Education Online, http://www.med-ed-online.org/res00023.htm).

ABOUT THE AUTHOR

His friends teased him mercilessly … "Don't go to his house for lunch … his mother will feed you meatless hotdogs and carrot juice!" Then there was the time the high-school principle told him to stay home for a few days because of the overwhelming odor of garlic emanating from his torso … Brent had had a cold, and phoned his mom in her health food store at the Bonnie Doon Shopping Center to ask what to do for it. She told him to take some garlic, so he enthusiastically gobbled up a large quantity, placing the cloves between slices of whole wheat bread. He never did hear the end of that one!

A few years later Brent left his parent's home in Edmonton, resolved not to have anything more to do with "health foods" and all the other nonsense that his mother tried to stuff him with. But an ever-present infatuation with the subject of nutrition continued to dog him, and his interest peaked anew when he had his own babies to care for, and wanted to give them the best nutrition possible. Without really knowing it, Brent had embarked on a life-long search for objective and unbiased knowledge about nutrition.

Just before his mother died in 1986, she sat down with him and talked about nutrition. She was a very disappointed woman at that time … she had devoted most of her life to learning about nutrition, and trying to help people with her knowledge. But her success had been limited … every single cancer sufferer she had worked with finally died of cancer, and her own health had always been a problem, starting with diabetes when she was just a young girl. But she over-flowed with tremendous faith, and tried to pass some of it on to her son. His mother suggested that he go back to university and apply his learning skills to the field of nutrition. She re-iterated what he already knew … that the field of nutrition, at least in Canada and the U.S., was starkly divided into two opposing camps. On one side was nutrition as formally studied in the universities and copyrighted by the medical doctors and professional dietitians and nutritionists. The other was the world of 'health foods' and supplements and alternative medicine. But Kathryn Bateman had a vision. She told Brent that there *was* a middle road … that yes, there was a lot of misinformation and nonsense … on both sides … but that a more correct nutritional perspective lay somewhere in-between, and she challenged her son to re-enter the ivory towers and seek that middle path.

So he did just that, but found himself struggling an up-hill battle. He learned very quickly that having grown up in a health food store was not something to brag about, and that it was best to keep his insights from that exposure a secret. But it eventually leaked out, and, combined with his outspokenness and questioning attitude, his academic ambitions suffered. First, he was refused continued study at the University of Hawaii in the master's program in nutrition, although he had earned top grades in the undergraduate program in the same department, and had already been in the master's program one full semester. It was apparent that it had a lot to do with his proposed thesis topic, which was to create a computer program to test the paradigm statement that "you can obtain all your required nutrients by eating a variety of basic foods and maintaining a balanced diet". This was viewed as an unsuitable topic for a student wishing to gain membership to the nutritionist's exclusive 'club'. A number of other criticisms had surfaced. Brent had been the student editor of the FSHN Newsletter, and had been outspoken. In his editorials he had dared to question some of the basic tenets of the conventional wisdom in nutrition and modern medicine. In class Brent had once objected to milk as "the perfect food" and had mentioned a study, just published, that something in cow's milk caused an auto-immune reaction which caused T-cells to attack the beta cells in the pancreas. His professor had told him that, quite frankly, he was "nuts". For one of his presentations he chose the study by Eaton and Konner of the Paleolithic diet. Then, the newly appointed advisor to the post-graduate acceptance committee was stanchly against supplements of any kind, and Brent had spoken up in his undergraduate class in favor of supplements. Although Brent received an "A" in that class, the professor made it clear that his pro-supplement attitude was "unacceptable". He was then told by this gentleman's close colleague that he "should choose another field of study".

Maybe being forced to leave the University of Hawaii program was a blessing, because Brent then discovered the Institute of Nutrition at Mahidol University in Thailand … an institute with a truly international perspective and curriculum, and a prestigious reputation. Ironically, he made this discovery via the same professor that told him he should seek another field of study. Brent was more careful this round, however, and chose a different thesis topic … and was very hush-hush about his experiences at the University of Hawaii, and his distant health food past. The director of the institute, and Brent's mentor, Dr. Kraisid Tontisirin, had known that Brent also possessed a B.A. in Economics, and suggested that his thesis combine economics and nutrition. Brent followed his advice, entitling the thesis "Nutriton Intervention: A Potential Factor For Economic Growth and Development". It was a great topic. But Dr. Kraisid left INMU shortly after Brent started on his thesis, becoming the director of the Food Policy and Nutrition Division of the FAO, stationed in Rome. Brent was required to find another advisor, and was passed from professor to professor; ending up with … wouldn't you believe it … a professor who was a good friend of his antagonist at the University of Hawaii … they had studied and received their PhD's together at Cornell. Once again he was under fire.

163

One of Brent's good friends, also from UH, coached him to be steadfast and to persevere. He re-wrote that 200 page thesis, end-to-end, fifteen separate times ... and it took three years of relentless effort. On the final day, after having successfully defended the thesis and meeting with his advisor for one last time ... she asked Brent what he wanted to do ... what were his plans. Brent told her he wanted to continue to study nutrition, and to write about nutrition. Her face darkened. She said "Brent, I know you '*come from the other side*'. I hope you don't write anything to hurt us." To this day Brent wonders at that statement, and all its implications, and is amazed that it was made by a PhD professor in nutrition.

During the frequent empty spaces of time, waiting for his Mahidol thesis advisor to review his latest version and tell him to re-write it once again, Brent travelled throughout Thailand, exploring every corner. He fell in love with the picturesque town of Sangkhlaburi, located at the northern end of the Khao Laem lake in Kanchanaburi Province, near the Myanmar border. He was astonished to see that there were no boats on the lake, so decided to make Sangkhlaburi his new home and capitalize on his life-long passion for boat-building. Brent encourages the reader to visit his website at www.sanghaleicanoeandkayak.com. Besides taking care of his boat shop and writing, Brent is involved in several other projects and has also found new directions to explore in nutrition and human health. One dream is to continue studying in a university setting ... the University of Chulalongkhan offers a PhD curriculum for international students in Public Health, with a specialty in nutrition. Brent is also working with a group of ethnic Mon and Karen to learn about the vast diversity of plants used by the indigenous peoples of Thailand and Myanmar, and is putting together a book in an attempt to preserve their vulnerable knowledge. He is also deeply interested in Thai Traditional Medicine. Who knows ... he may one day open a health/nutrition spa in his hide-away home alongside the beautiful Khao Laem lake.

www.ingramcontent.com/pod-product-compliance
Lightning Source LLC
Chambersburg PA
CBHW050123280326
41933CB00010B/1226